In Horizontal Orbit

*Hospitals and
the Cult of Efficiency*

In Horizontal Orbit

Hospitals and
the Cult of Efficiency

CAROL TAYLOR

University of Florida

HOLT, RINEHART AND WINSTON

New York   Chicago   San Francisco   Atlanta
Dallas   Montreal   Toronto   London   Sydney

for DOROTHY M. SMITH

*To whom nursing is not only a way of life
but also a way into life.*

Preface

This book deals with the various ways in which our society organizes itself to delay death, defeat disease, and seek health. It emerged from a ten-year study centralized in the medical center that introduced decentralized management into the contemporary hospital, and it is dedicated to the person who made this significant change possible. Its title *In Horizontal Orbit* is a comment on the curious way in which our health systems, both public and private, reduce patients to an inferior status. This phenomenon is most visible in the hospital where the two health systems overlap. It is most striking when the patient is being shuttled on a hospital stretcher from one part of the building to another.

In Horizontal Orbit was written for students in all health-related professions, and it is intended to make visible the dynamics of the social systems within which students will function when they become doctors, nurses, hospital administrators, and the like. It is written from the point of view of the outside-insider: an observer who, like the poet in the Middle Ages, watched the battle in order to write about it, but did not otherwise participate.

The first part is about the hospital, the second part is about the roles and relationships of the hospital's patient and working populations, and the last one consists of a brief glance at the society that produced this institution and these relationships. *In Horizontal Orbit* introduces the reader to a number of different topics and in some cases these topics cannot be handled in depth. Notes about the theory relevant to each of the three parts are to be found at the end of the text.

Gainesville, Fla.   C. T.
September 1969

Acknowledgments

When one takes a decade examining a process before writing a book about it, those persons to whom one is obligated have become too numerous to mention by name. I owe a special debt of gratitude to those who encouraged me to take a long and intimate look at the hospital culture, and to those who assisted me in writing *In Horizontal Orbit*. Dorothy Smith enabled me to take a long look at the hospital culture, and Samuel Martin and Esther Lucille Brown encouraged me to do so. Hannah Kimball edited early drafts of the manuscript in such a way as to nudge my writing into some sort of style. Alice and Clyde Murphree provided me with a place to work when I most desperately needed it. Gwen Neville helped at a critical point in the preparation of the manuscript, and David P. Boynton tolerated inordinate delays during the revisions of it. My husband, Griffin Taylor, and our daughters, Anne and Mary, made it possible for me to begin and to finish the book.

I also wish to thank *Nursing Forum* and the *American Journal of Nursing* for permission to republish materials included in Chapter 7.

Contents

In Horizontal Orbit

Hospitals and
the Cult of Efficiency

Part   One

THE HOSPITAL

1

Looking at Hospitals

In a technically sophisticated society such as ours, the care of the sick is most conspicuous when it is concentrated in the hospital. For this reason, I began my examination of the various ways in which our society organizes itself to seek health, to defeat disease, and to delay death, by looking at the hospital. Before I looked at one, I made a note of previous experiences that might predispose me to see what I expected rather than what I was looking at. The following extracts from my field diary suggest what my biases were when I began to examine hospitals in October 1958:

> The hospital belongs to a group of institutions with which I am familiar, the large-scale organization. Previous studies have left a significant bias: I find distasteful some of the ways in which large-scale organizations impose institutionalized roles.

This bias showed when I compared the hospital's admission process with brainwashing—fortunately, this comparison was productive.

I had two experiences at the hospital as a patient not in critical condition: I gave birth to a baby in one hospital and had my appendix removed in another.

During the first experience, I refused to submit to the institution's decision that all patients admitted to deliver babies were not to be fed until they had done so. A medically sound decision for those in labor, but one which I considered inappropriate for a patient like myself who had been taken into the hospital before the onset of labor. My physician was not present to arbitrate; and when I consumed a meal intended for another patient, I became, as one nurse put it, "the worst patient this hospital has ever had."

During the second experience, my decision to act in what I considered a common sense manner earned me the good-patient label.

The gadget the hospital had provided to permit me to listen to piped-in music broke down and I fixed it with my nail file. When the nurse saw what I was doing, she brought me three others to repair. News of my ability to tighten screws spread, and I was loaned a screwdriver and given the opportunity to repair speakers from other parts of the hospital. During this hospital stay I was complimented and given special privileges.

The contrast between these two experiences suggested a question that I later attempted to answer. For what reasons are patients labeled "good" and "bad"?

My single experience at the hospital as a patient in critical condition included the following incident:

While two surgeons were stitching my head, one stopped and said: "It's a complete waste of time. She's going to die." I tried to say: "I'm going to live, get on with the job."

The consequence of this experience was an interest in finding the answer to two questions. How frequently do patients overhear comments obviously not intended for their ears? This was a question for which I found an answer. I also wondered whether or not the patient who thinks he may die gives up and dies when a remark like this is made over his apparently unconscious body. I could think of no satisfactory way to answer this question, but I decided to ask it in case the answer is yes. The asking of it has had interesting consequences.

My previous experiences as a patient-visitor were limited, and I summed them up with the following comment:

Visiting rules and regulations seem unduly restrictive, but it is possible to find nurses who are prepared to wink an eye at their infringement.

This comment suggested an interesting question. Do nurses and others who work in hospitals use the opportunity either to enforce or to modify the institution's rules and regulations as a reward and punishment system?

From time to time I had worked as a volunteer in hospitals, on three occasions in an unusual capacity. I summed up these experiences by noting:

> Despite the circumstances that precipitated three of them, these experiences should make me feel comfortable in a hospital rather than biased about the treatment patients receive.

After recording my experiences with hospitals as accurately as possible, I began to look at one to see if I could discover how it functioned.

One of my first observations was that the persons encountered during this examination made interesting and, in some cases, surprising comments about hospitals. This observation suggested a collection of comments about hospitals. The following sample, collected during a three day visit to New York in 1960, is characteristic of what I found when I listened to what others said about hospitals:

> The man behind the hotel desk told me that a particular hospital was famous for its operations, and suggested that I visit it. The elevator operator described that same hospital as a place where "they experiment on people," and advised me to try another where "they let you die in peace." And the bellhop said: "I don't want to have anything to do with hospitals and that's for sure."

> The taxicab driver said: "I was born in one, and I guess I'll die in one."

> A seven-year-old boy said: "I was born in this hospital, and now they're going to take out my tonsils."

> A thirty-seven-year-old man said: "My wife and I haven't needed a hospital since the kids were born, thank God. My brother-in-law was here when they cut off his leg, and now my father is upstairs dying of cancer. They do the best they can for you, but it is no place for a man to be."

> A man and his wife explained that they were coming in for their annual checkup, and the man said: "We don't spare expense when it comes to health."

> A woman with purple hair said: "My sister-in-law is upstairs bragging about the surgeon that took out her appendix. I use hospital X. Three years ago a team of their surgeons took out nearly everything I had."

> A waitress said: "They work hard in hospitals, but they get interesting cases. The doctors and nurses from across the street come in to eat, and when we're not too busy, I polish tables and listen to them talk about their work. You'd be surprised at what they do over there."

"Over there" those who did these surprising things made these comments:

> The woman at the information desk said: "This is my third hospital, and our problem is that hospitals are full of information this desk is not

allowed to give out, and sometimes the public get rude about it. Today, we have a chronic—the father of a lady in labor. He calls every hour on the hour. He was at it all night, and he has telephoned three times since I came on. The last time when I said: "Mrs. so-and-so has not had her baby yet, but she's struggling nobly," which is what this desk is supposed to say, he said: "She's been struggling nobly for eleven hours. How long does it take to have a baby for gosh sakes?"

A candy striper summed up the hospital as "an exciting place to work, but you do have sad experiences," and she described one.

A nursing supervisor described the hospital as "a place where nurses care for patients while doctors work on them."

A physician said: "As far as I am concerned, the best hospital is the hospital with the best facilities."

A floor nurse said: "A hospital is a place where you work your tail off." Another added: "We're overworked and underpaid, but don't knock it. Every time a hopeless case recovers, it's more than worth it."

An aide said: "You get a chance to help people. That's why I'm here, which is more than I can say for some I could name."

And a hospital administrator ended his explanation of the hospital by saying: "As you can see, hospitals are one of the biggest industries in the country."

These opinions and others like them do not add up to a description of the hospital. They reflect individual experiences with hospitals, and they tell us something about the different ways in which people think and feel about hospitals.

To its potential customers, the hospital seems to be a number of different things. A place to die in peace, and a place where death is fought. Where one is born, and where one seeks health. It also is a place where more or less spectacular operations are undergone and, in some cases, boasted about. To those who work in it, the hospital seems somewhat different. To the physician, it is a convenient and necessary facility. To the administrator, it is a business that survives even when it loses money. To the nurse, it is a place where, however hard she works, the work is never done. But, as one nurse reminded us, "When a hopeless case recovers, it's more than worth it." And most of those who work in hospitals would agree that the hospital provides a way of life which is both frustrating and extremely rewarding.

While I was collecting the comments that suggested these points of view, I also was examining the hospital as a social system; and I will devote the rest of this chapter to making the hospital visible as a social system. There are a number of different ways in which social systems can be made visible enough to study. When I examine one, I begin by diagraming the way in which it has organized itself to function. As soon as this skeleton has been completed, I look at the processes that give structure its purpose; in short, I watch the system as it works. Some social systems are small enough to be examined as totalities while others must be examined part by part and put together again before they can be seen as a dynamic whole. The hospital must be examined part by part and put together again before it can be understood as one system.

Where does one begin to study a complex social system like the hospital? A satisfactory start could be made by examining any part of it, but I prefer to look first at the part that does what the system has been organized to do. A hospital is organized to care for sick persons while cures are attempted, and I began my study of it by looking at the patient-care units. First, I diagramed the formal structure of each unit. This information was readily available on organization charts. Next, I began to observe on these units, and I looked first for information confirming and contradicting the institution's notion of how it had organized itself to function. The following extracts from my field diary suggest the type of information that emerged when I approached the in-patient units in this manner:

> The organization chart places Mr. A, Dr. B, and Miss C at the same level in the hierarchy, and it seems to expect them to function as peers. (Mr. A was the administrator of a sixty-four bed unit; Dr. B was the physician in charge, and Miss C was the nurse in charge.) During my initial interviews with these three persons, they described their responsibilities and decision-making rights in such a way as to indicate that all three of them functon and relate to each other in exactly the way the organization chart suggests. However, they made comments about each other which led me to suspect that they have reorganized themselves in a somewhat different manner.

> Dr. B said that Miss C was "a jewel," and that Mr. A was "alright as long as he is kept busy."

> Miss C said: "Dr. B and I understand each other. Mr. A's boss does not understand, and sometimes couldn't care less about, the problems on the unit."

> Mr. A said: "It's a privilege to work with doctors," and "I don't know how the floor would run without Miss C."

I began to observe Mr. A at work. After doing so for two weeks, I recorded the following comments:

> Observations show that Mr. A spends two to three hours each day providing services for individual physicians. He runs errands for them, composes and types their letters, makes telephone calls for them, and

does not seem upset when a passing physician takes the pen out of his hand and walks off with it.

When I talked with Mr. A about his relationship with the physicians, he said: "They appreciate what I do for them. Dr. X liked the way I rearranged their conference room," and "It is a privilege associating with doctors."

During my observations of Mr. A at work, it became obvious that Miss C made decisions about what supplies should be ordered, how the budget was to be used, and about what Mr. A's clerical staff were to do. (In formal interviews with me both Mr. A and Miss C had confirmed the chart's statement that decisions of this sort were made by Mr. A.)

Mr. A said about Miss C, "She takes a load off me."

And the comments of Mr. A's staff suggest that they recognize Miss C as Mr. A's boss. They were heard saying to each other such things as: "You'd better not do it until you ask Miss C. Miss C said to go ahead. Mr. A did not know that Miss C wanted it done this way."

My emerging conclusion was that Miss C had placed Mr. A in a position subordinate to herself, and that Mr. A accepts this arrangement although he may not realize that his position in the hierarchy has shifted. I wondered what happened when Mr. A's boss ordered him to do something that either Dr. B or Miss C took exception to.

I collected a number of examples of what happened when Mr. A's boss made unpopular decisions. The one below was selected because, in addition to showing us what happens, it is an example of the way in which physicians use their own rules when they play the bureaucratic game:

Yesterday, Mr. A's boss decided that suture sets were to be signed out by the physicians who used them. (Mr. A's boss later explained that he made this decision because he was "determined to decrease the loss of scissors.") Today, I concentrated on the surgical units knowing that their frequent need to take out stitches would make them most irritated with the new procedure.

On Mr. A's floor I heard a number of surgeons complain to Dr. B about signing out suture sets. In each case Dr. B said: "So, forget it. I'll talk to Miss C and we'll fix it." On one occasion he added, "Don't blame A, its that front office so-and-so."

I was in Miss C's office when Dr. B talked with her about signing out suture sets. He said: "It's ridiculous, my men haven't the time for it." She said: "Poor A gets caught in the middle." He said: "How do you want to handle it?" And she said: "Why don't you go down and blow your stack." Dr. B left, presumably to blow his stack in so-and-so's front office.

The following extract from my field diary suggests that Dr. B's violation of correct communication channels, going over A's head and behind his own boss's back, was effective:

> When I arrived on the floor at ten o'clock this morning (the following day), the suture sign-out sheet was not in evidence. Some hours later, in the middle of a conversation about the steps that were being taken to rid the unit of cockroaches, Mr. A said: "Dr. B is a great guy, he sure goes to bat for us."

This sequence shows how Mr. A, Dr. B, and Miss C reorganized themselves to function in a manner somewhat different from that described in the organization chart.

Further examination showed other interesting rearrangements: Those responsible to Miss C and those responsible through others to her did not, in all cases, function according to the organization chart. Dr. B's men (seven men and one woman) also had organized into an informal system somewhat different from that described by the chart. And, as we saw earlier, Mr. A's staff acted as if they were responsible through Mr. A to Miss C. I found that all patient-care units in the hospital had reorganized themselves to function in ways other than those suggested by the organization chart. And the fascinating thing about these rearrangements was that no two of them were exactly alike.

According to the organization chart the patient-care units were organized in one way, but according to my observations other and somewhat different organizational systems existed and functioned vigorously. On each unit I began to look at these two systems—the formal system described by the organization chart and the informal system I had observed—as if they were two horses harnessed to the same wagon. It soon became obvious that unless the two systems had compatible objectives, the informal system was able to defeat the intentions of the formal system—the skirmish about signing out suture sets was a case in point.

In order to understand why these informal systems developed, we need some understanding of the formal system. The hospital is organized and administered in a bureaucratic manner, but it differs from a classical bureaucracy in one respect: two of its specialists, the physician and the nurse, break the rules of the bureaucratic game whenever the needs of their patients make it seem necessary to do so. The physician because he thinks of the hospital as a facility to be used for the benefit of his patients does not think it necessary, in all instances, to go through the hospital's formal channels of communication and command. Consequently, he speaks his mind to maids, to maintenance men, to floor nurses, and to administrators whenever it seems desirable to do so. The nurse is responsible for seeing to it that the needs of the hospital's patients are met, and because these needs arise at night, during weekends, on Christmas day, and at other times when service departments are closed, she invades these alien territories in order to satisfy the most urgent needs of her patients. As a consequence the nurse periodically acts as if she were a pharmacist, a dietitian, a sterile-supply worker, a maid, and a storekeeper. These organizational peculiarities will be examined after we have taken a look at a classical bureaucratic system.

A bureaucratic system is a logical attempt to see to it that the idiosyncrasies of individuals do not interfere with a large-scale organization's ability to accomplish a specific task, and it usually is diagramed as a system of offices [1] (Fig. 1).

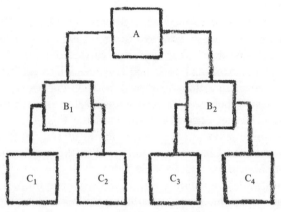

Figure 1.

In such a system, decision-making is centralized toward the top of the pyramid, and other kinds of work are decentralized toward its base. In the miniature system presented above, A decides what B_1 and B_2 are supposed to do. Then B_1 makes a similar decision for C_1 and C_2, while B_2 does the same for C_3 and C_4. The four C's are supposed to do what they are told to do and to do it as directed. In a system organized and administered in this manner, communication through correct channels (B_1 through A to B_2) protects the decision-making rights vested in each office and sees to it that the functions which differentiate one office from another remain stable. It is obvious that the physician's communication pattern and the nurse's habit of expanding and contracting her functional responsibilities interfere with the hospital's ability to behave in a bureaucratic manner.[2]

[1] For an analysis of the elegant logic of the bureaucratic system, *see* Max Weber, *The Theory of Social and Economic Organization,* trans. A. M. Henderson and T. Parsons (New York: The Free Press, 1947).

[2] For a detailed description, *see* H. L. Smith, "Two Lines of Authority" in *Patients, Physicians, and Illness,* E. G. Jaco ed. (New York: The Free Press, 1958), pp. 468–477; 3d ed. (1963), 448–467.

The informal organization and action that tend to develop in all bureaucratic systems, including hospitals, characteristically serve two purposes. At middle levels in the hierarchy they by-pass formal channels of communication and command to permit cooperative action which either makes the operation less cumbersome or modifies decisions made at higher levels. Dr. B and Miss C worked together in this manner, and in the system drawn above, B_1 and B_2 would tend to develop an informal working relationship that would serve the same purpose. At the lowest level in a bureaucratic system, in our diagram the four C's, informal action is taken. Its purpose is to set limits on the system's ability to make demands that are considered either unreasonable or unjust. In a system organized to produce inanimate objects, a sausage factory for example, this informal action is facilitated by those directly responsible for overseeing the lowest level workers. In a system organized to process people—hospitals, schools, prisons, and so forth—those at the lowest level in the formal system tend to incorporate those who are being processed into their system of informal action. They develop a set of rewards and punishments that enables them to meet what otherwise might be unrealistic expectations on the part of the institution. Prisons and state mental hospitals are excellent places to look for this phenomenon.

Hospitals, until they began to experiment with decentralized management, were bureaucratic systems into which two organizational peculiarities had been assimilated: the roving communication pattern of the physician and the shifting functions of the nurse. The suture-set skirmish, described earlier in this chapter, is an example of what happens when both informal bureaucratic behavior and the behavior that distinguishes hospitals from other bureaucratic systems are present. Both Dr. B and Miss C felt that Mr. A did not function effectively, presumably because his boss "didn't understand, and sometimes couldn't care less about, the problems on the unit." Mr. A, Dr. B, and Miss C rearranged matters so that Mr. A stayed in the background, while Dr. B and Miss C worked together to change decisions made by Mr. A's boss when they felt that it was to the best interest of the unit to do so. Such informal action can be found in most bureaucratic systems. The way in which Miss C and Dr. B attacked the unpopular decision that suture sets were to be signed out also reflects the characteristic behavior which distinguishes hospitals from other kinds of bureaucratic systems. The nurse's habit of shifting from one function to another encouraged Miss C to make decisions that were not being made and implemented in a satisfactory manner by Mr. A, an administrator. And it seemed perfectly natural to Dr. B, a physician, that she should do so. Mr. A may not have realized, and certainly did not appear to resent, the way in which his authority has been diminished. Mr. A's boss may have been unaware of the true state of affairs. Dr. B periodically told him that Mr. A was "doing a good job," and on the rare occasions when Mr.

A's boss visited the floor, Mr. A seemed to be in command of administrative matters.

The physician, even when he is on the hospital payroll, does not play the bureaucratic game in quite the same way that it is played by other categories of hospital worker. Everyone, including the physician, uses the informal system to modify the intent of the formal system to fit specific situations and needs. Everyone, except the physician, does so in such a way as to make it seem as if the bureaucratically correct channels of communication and command have been used. The physician is the only one in the hospital who feels free to speak his mind to persons at all levels in the hierarchy. When it seems necessary, the physician rebukes the maid, a person who does not work for him; and confronts the hospital director who is the manager of the system in which he, the physician, works. Also he does not feel that he is going "behind backs" and "over heads" when he communicates in this manner. Consequently, it did not seem strange to those concerned when Dr. B went to Mr. A's boss to "blow his stack." When Dr. B asked Miss C "How do you want to handle it?" he was asking her whether she wanted to take it up through channels, report the problem to *her* front office, or whether she wanted him to use his freedom to question the unpopular decision in a more direct manner.

While I was observing the formal and informal organization and action on the patient-care units, I began to notice interesting contradictions between what people said they were doing and what they actually were doing. The following observations show what I found, and how I used what I found.

The nurse in charge of one unit was interrupted during an interview in which she was explaining her nursing philosophy to a visiting researcher and the following exchanges were recorded:

> Nurse in charge to visitor: "The most important thing is to remember that the patient is a person. I devote considerable in-service time (a continuing education program) to this particular topic. My aim is to get rid of the bedside manner, the how-are-we-this-morning approach, and see to it that the care of each patient on my unit is personalized." A staff nurse knocks on the partly open door and sticks her head around it. She said: "Mrs. D in 604 keeps insisting that she needs a painkiller, and I can't do anything with her." Nurse in charge to staff nurse: "Give her a placebo. When you've settled 604, give the colostomy in 615 a sitz bath."

This interchange suggested two questions. How do nurses and other hospital specialists acknowledge the fact that the patient is a person? When, how, and by whom is he treated like a thing? The following entry in my diary describes the circumstances in which I discovered one clue to the answers I sought:

Had lunch with seven nurses. They talked at considerable length about their patients, and I was fascinated to notice that three of them invariably referred to their patients by diagnostic label—the craniotomy, the skull fracture, and so forth. The other four talked about these same patients as if they were people. They did not use names, presumably because they were talking about confidential matters in a public place, instead they used descriptive phrases—sweet old lady, just a kid, nice guy but weird, and so forth. I wonder if there is a relationship between a nurse's habit of talking about her patient as a person and her ability to treat him like one? Observations of these seven nurses at work and interviews with their patients might be profitable.

My observations supported the notion that such a relationship existed, and subsequent talks with patients seemed to confirm it. A chance observation suggested another possibility:

While I was talking to Dr. X (a radiologist), I saw Mr. L spring to his feet, and say: "I am a right elbow." (Mr. L was a patient who had told me that he "absolutely refused to be treated like a piece of furniture by anyone in the hospital.") Some hours later I encountered Mr. L, and he said: "Most extraordinary thing happened. Went to x-ray. Handed the request form to a girl at a desk; she was talking to a boyfriend on the phone. Sat down and began to wait. Ten minutes later an old lady came in and did the same thing. She (the old lady) coughed and spat into a bottle every five minutes or so—obvious chest case. The boyfriend got off the line and the girl called a girl friend. Twenty minutes later the girl hung up, got to her feet, and went through a door with both request slips in her hand. Three minutes later she came back with one request slip, leaned against the wall and looked at it. Then she raised her head, and looked at the two of us, a woman coughing into a bottle and a man with his arm in a sling, and said: "Who is the right elbow?" To my surprise I sprang to my feet, and claimed to be the elbow she was looking for. It's unbelievable. The system keeps me waiting fifty-seven minutes, then it addresses me as something less than human, and what do I do? Leap to my feet and claim to be a right elbow." I left Mr. L's room wondering to what extent patients aid and abet the hospital as it dehumanizes them."

During my examination of the patient-care units, I began to collect telephone conversations with service departments. The first observation in this sequence describes the interchange that awakened my interest in the relationship between patient-care units and the departments that service them:

A nurse was talking about how hospitals have changed: "You used to be able to pick up the phone and tell them (service departments) to do it or else. Now we have to handle them with velvet gloves." A physician approached and said: "There are no scissors on the treatment tray."

> A clerk called Sterile Supply and, after a considerable argument about who was at fault, said: "What do you expect us to do, take them out with our teeth?"

I used the following observation to sum up this particular sequence:

> At 10:30 A.M., the administrator of unit P said: "I've sent six orders to maintenance, and the bathroom door is still off its hinges." At 11:30 A.M., I was in the office of the administrator of unit Q when a man in a maintenance uniform stuck his head through the doorway and asked: "Anything need fixing today?"

Contrasts of this type led me into the service departments to see what patient-care units looked like from their point of view. And from these departments I moved into other parts of the hospital in order to examine all the departments that directly or indirectly support the central function of the hospital which is to diagnose, to treat, and to care for patients.

In each part of the hospital I did what I had done in the patient-care units: I began with structure, both formal and informal; and then examined the processes that gave the structure its purpose. In order to do so, I looked for four kinds of information. Information confirming and contradicting the institution's notion of how it had organized each of its parts to function. Information about how each part did, or did not do, whatever it was supposed to do. Information about what the people who worked in each department actually do and about what they said they were doing, as well as information about each department's functional relationship with various departments and other parts of the hospital. In all parts of the hospital, I found that the people in each part had organized themselves to function in ways that were different from those suggested by the organization chart. I also found that individuals described what they did, and what their departments did, in such a way as to contradict what I could observe being done. In a sense my study of the hospital was patterned on the contradictions that I found in it.

When I had examined all parts of the hospital in this manner, I looked for the first time at the hospital as a dynamic whole, and I checked my understanding of it by returning and observing each part of the hospital as a part of this whole. When I had made minor corrections, and was satisfied that I had a working understanding of the various ways in which the hospital actually behaved, I began to place it in social context and historical perspective. In order to do so, I began to look at and think about such things as:

(1) the various professions to which hospital specialists belong and the ways in which each of these professions is organized to discharge its responsibilities to society;

(2) the history of the institutions, professions, and problems that I had found in the hospital; and

(3) the changes in our society that might require the hospital to make changes.

This kind of information places the hospital in social context as a dynamic part of a changing society, and helped me to understand it. I will use some historical information about the hospital to suggest how new insights emerge when this is done.

As its name suggests, the hospital began as a place in which a community discharged its responsibility for offering hospitality to passing strangers. Before it was transplanted to this continent, the hospital had become a place where the community discharged another responsibility: to care for those of its members who were unable to care for themselves. A rapid increase in the size of communities precipitated the separation of community members needing care into specialized institutions, and by the turn of the century the city hospital in this country had become a place where the critically ill and the dying poor were cared for. In less densely populated areas all categories of the materially resourceless were placed in "poor farms" unless they were able to work, in which case the responsibility of caring for them was contracted out to the highest bidder.[3] Vestiges of the peonage system produced by this practice persisted into the 1920s.

The arbitrariness with which hospitals tend to treat their patients becomes more understandable when one realizes that, until relatively recently, hospital patients could have been sold into peonage if they had not been too ill to work. Florida, for example, outlawed peonage in the early nineteen twenties.[4] During the last quarter of the nineteenth century, the Elizabethan style of assuming responsibility for the care of the "poor," and those otherwise handicapped, was being replaced by a system of custodial care designed to protect persons in these categories from exploitation. Until relatively recently, custodial care was considered desirable. It is now thought of as "not good enough" and the word "custodial" has been stigmatized. At the turn of the present century, the hospital was a place where poor people died, and the role of hospital patient was intended for persons who were in critical condition and had become a financial burden to society. At that time dominant segments of the society tended to equate material success with "godliness."

During the present century, the status of the hospital has changed rapidly for a number of reasons. A recognition of the need for asceptic

---

[3] This practice stemmed from the Elizabethan poor law.

[4] This case is documented in the archives of the General Extension Division, Florida State University System.

techniques and a sterile field during childbirth and surgery brought operations and birth out of the home into the hospital. Advances in medical knowledge and rapid technological development made the hospital an increasingly attractive facility. And the Depression of the Thirties expanded the hospital's patient-population to include many persons who previously would have hired nurses to care for them in their homes. It also moved the nurse out of the community into the hospital. During the first half of the present century, the hospital changed from a place where poor people died to a place where most of us are born, are subjected to elaborate checkups, undergo surgery, are treated for certain diseases, and eventually may die.[5]

The patient and those who work with the patient have been critically affected by these changes, in some cases to the benefit of those concerned, and in other cases adversely. The physician has emerged with an opportunity to use expensive facilities and services for the benefit of his patients. Those with an administrative turn of mind have acquired an opportunity to run a business that is expected to lose money. The nurse has become a hospital employee with the consequence that she is torn between her traditional responsibilities for the patient and her new responsibilities to the hospital. A large number of new specialties have emerged, and as a consequence the hospital has become an extremely complex social system. The patient has profited by advances in medical knowledge and technology, but some measure of this gain has been eroded by the hospital's tendency to dehumanize him. In addition, the community has acquired a facility it needs, but cannot decide how to pay for. These gains and losses will be examined in considerable detail in succeeding chapters. They are mentioned here to suggest the way in which *In Horizontal Orbit* grew out of the process demonstrated in this chapter.

The process examined in this book is one that does things to and for people. The book's title *In Horizontal Orbit* comments on a characteristic common to all people-processing systems in our society. When we organize ourselves to do things to and for people—educate them, cure them, care for them, and so forth—we tend to use what I think of as conveyor-belt logic. An excellent approach to the task of producing nuts, bolts, sausages, and other inanimate objects, but one with obvious pitfalls when the object to be processed is animate and human. Consequently, our people-processing systems tend to expect more conveyor-belt behavior than is absolutely necessary, and those persons being processed characteristically draw attention to this fact by sporadic refusals to conform to

[5] For a more explicit statement about this change, *see* G. Rosen, "The Hospital: Historical Sociology of a Community Institution," in *The Hospital In Modern Society: Eleven Studies of the Hospital Today,* E. Freidson, ed. (New York: The Free Press, 1963), 1–36.

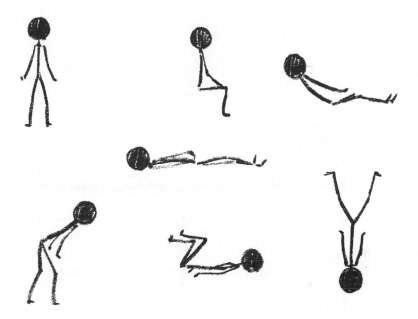

Figure 2. Positioning systems used by health specialists.

particular demands. Recent suits against school systems that refuse to teach the long-haired male is an excellent example.

As far as our health systems are concerned, skirmishes of this type tend to focus on the way in which the body of the patient is prepared for and positioned during diagnosis, treatment, and care. Patients ask:

"Why do I have to eat in bed when I'm allowed to sit in a chair?"

"Why do I have to undress and get into bed if they aren't going to do anything to me until tomorrow?"

"Why do I have to be wheeled about when I am perfectly capable of walking?"

"Did whoever invented this contraption (the wheel used during a sigmoidscopy) realize what it feels like to be examined by a bunch of doctors when you're stood on your head?" [6]

Comments voicing similar complaints can be collected in physicians' offices, clinics, and public health departments:

"Why must I strip to the waist to have my ears washed out?"

[6] I have been told that from a technological point of view, the "wheel" facilitates a sigmoidscopy because it straightens out the gut.

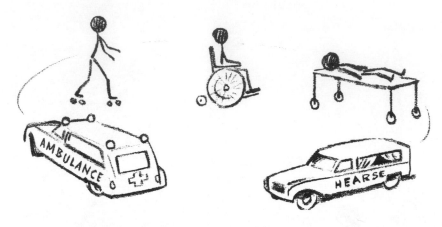

Figure 3.

"Why can't they schedule appointments so that you don't have to wait two hours?"

"It takes all day to get 'the pill.' They (the public health nurses) lecture you all morning, keep you hanging about while they take their time eating, do 'the smear' and, after another long wait, you get the paper that gets you 'the pill'."

For the most part patients do not refuse to eat in bed, strip to the waist, or be wheeled about when they can walk, and they do attend the lecture and permit the Pap smear in order to get "the pill." But a surprising number of them object to these excessive demands. A patient who had been flat on his back during most of a hospital stay summed up his experiences by saying, "I usually confront bureaucracies in a vertical rather than a horizontal position."

It seemed to me that this comment was particularly apt, and my title *In Horizontal Orbit* emerged as a response to it. *Horizontal* because this position is the central one in the positioning system used by those in the health professions; (Fig, 2) and *In Orbit* to suggest that during the course of diagnosis, treatment, and care, patients, both in the hospital and out of it, are programmed into irregularly, eliptical journeys within buildings and from building to building (Fig. 3).

2

Conflicting Frames of Reference

A by-product of one of the changes mentioned toward the end of the last chapter, the increase in different kinds of specialized workers, has increased the potential for friction among hospital workers. When differently specialized people are brought together into the same system, one frequently finds what I call "conflicting frames of reference." In a hospital culture these conflicts sometimes interfere with the smooth running of the hospital, but they are extremely useful to anyone interested in understanding it as a social system. Frame-of-reference conflicts can be used by the observer to identify decision-making boundaries and to predict changes in decision-making territories. In this chapter, I am going to show three conflicting frames of reference by examining the characteristic responses of three categories of hospital specialists to one phenomenon: the patient's ability to pay his hospital bill. The three specialists are: the administrator, the physician, and the nurse.

The administrator is responsible, among other things, for keeping the hospital out of debt. He is delighted when patients can pay their hospital bills, and he is tempted to order "red carpet" treatment for those patients who might donate money to the hospital in addition to paying their bill. It is interesting that the term "red carpet" has become part of the hospital vocabulary. "Red carpet" treatment means showing special consideration to important persons, and it refers to the practice of carpeting the entrances to the hotel for royalty and for other distinguished visitors. The hospital vocabulary now includes many words borrowed from the hotel's vocabulary. The hospital's instructions about personalizing patient care are frequently expressed in words that one normally associates with hotels. The hospital reminds its employees that patients are people, and many of the words used for this purpose give one the impression that the hospital now thinks of itself as a specialized hotel. It is not uncommon to find sentences on hospital procedures that are inserted to remind the staff that the patient is the hospital's "guest."[1]

The physician has inherited the tradition of allowing the "rich" patient to contribute to the care of the "poor" patient. Special consideration for patients who are in a position to make substantial donations to the hospital, or for medical research, does not seem unreasonable to the physician. The phrase "red carpet" may seem inappropriate to the physician, but the practice of encouraging the "rich" patient to make a substantial donation to the hospital is not an alien concept to him.

The nurse's reactions to the patient's pay category are more complicated than the reactions of either the administrator or the physician. Like the administrator and the physician, the nurse believes that any sick person who needs care should receive care whether or not he can afford to pay for it. In addition, the nurse tends to resent the notion of "red carpet" treatment as a suggestion that she would give superior care to a patient merely because he could afford to pay for it. When the nurse is put in a situation in which the hospital seems to be asking her to skimp her care for a "poor" patient who is in critical condition in order to make special concessions to a "rich" patient who is not in desperate need of nursing care, she, the nurse, is apt to become resentful—and rightfully so.

The hospital administrator, the physician, and the nurse would all agree that any sick person in desperate need of hospital care should receive the best care available whether or not he can pay for it. The physician would tend to agree with the administrator about paying particular attention to an important patient. But, unless the administrator is extremely tactful, his suggestions about special care for special patients may be misinterpreted by the nurses, and his attempts to secure "red-carpet" treatment may misfire. If a hospital administrator really wants special consideration shown

[1] In 1829 The Tremont House in Boston introduced the practice of training hotel staff. One of the primary points made to trainees was that the hotel's "guests" were to be treated with dignity and respect, apparently a new concept at that time. The word "guest" on hospital procedures is supposed to convey the same message.

to an influential or wealthy patient, the most inept thing he can do is to seem to *order* Nursing Service to provide it: a fact that has been pointed out to me by a number of hospital administrators.

What happens when the hospital administrator seems to order Nursing Service to provide "red carpet" treatment? The hospital administrator asks the director of Nursing Service to see to it that her nurses give a particular patient special consideration. He explains to her why it is important for the hospital to make a good impression on this particular patient. The director of Nursing Service passes the order along through Nursing Service communication channels, and the order finally reaches the nurses who are expected to give "red carpet" treatment to a very important "guest."

Resistance begins to build up as soon as the order leaves the hospital administrator's office. The director of Nursing Service tends to resent the order as a criticism of her staff even when she agrees that it makes good business sense to pay special attention to this particular patient. As the order approaches the favored patient's bedside, the good business sense begins to disappear, and there is an increasing tendency to regard the order as a criticism of the nurses. As soon as this happens the nurse's latent resentment of the "rich" person's ability to buy hospital attention for insignificant complaints is mobilized. Even when the "red carpet" patient is in what the nurses consider a genuine state of "hospital sickness," it becomes increasingly difficult for the nurses to care for the patient without resenting him. When the "red carpet" patient is a woman, this process tends to be accelerated; when the "red carpet" patient is a child, particularly a young child, the latent resentment tends to remain dormant; and when it is a man the respective age of both nurse and patient become pertinent factors. What usually happens when sufficient resentment has been aroused is that formal "red carpet" treatment is given, and informal behavior sees to it that the "red carpet" treatment is sabotaged. I will use the first "red carpet" conflict that I observed, as an illustration:

> The patient told me that the nurses were giving him wonderful care. They always answered his bell promptly; they tried to get him what- ever he wanted; and they were meticulous in caring for him. When I asked him to describe the things about his hospital experience that were most frustrating to him, he listed four ways in which the life-style on the unit irritated him. He disliked being wakened and washed at six- o'clock in the morning. It made him feel disoriented not to be able to see the ground from his window. The wheels on hospital equipment made so much noise that it disturbed him, and he could not understand why the manufacturers did not do something about it. Although the nurses continually battled with Dietary on his behalf, he could not get an extra pot of coffee for breakfast. As he said, these were trivial irri- tations, and he was not complaining.

The interesting thing about these trivial irritations, however, was that they were either manufactured or they could have been eliminated. The traditional six o'clock waking and washing was not routine for all patients. On that unit at that particular time, the nurses were experimenting with the feasibility of letting patients who were asleep stay asleep until just before breakfast. Only those who already were awake were supposed to be washed as early as six o'clock in the morning.

The patient had to remain flat on his back, and from the usual bed-level he could not see the ground from his window. In an adjacent room a patient with a similar difficulty was routinely cranked up so that he could see from flat on *his* back the tops of trees and a distant rise of ground. I was puzzled by the mention of noisy wheels because this patient was at the dead end of a corridor, and I could not imagine that there would be sufficient traffic to justify his complaint. I assumed that he had sensitive ears.

A few days later, I saw something interesting. I was standing at the nursing station talking to a visitor when I saw a nurse dramatically change her behavior. She had been wheeling a blood pressure machine at a brisk walk in and out of the rooms and up the corridor toward the "red carpet" patient's room. Three doors away from the end of the corridor the nurse's behavior changed, she seemed in a tremendous hurry, and she ran out of one door through another door. When she finally reached the last door, the one behind which the "red carpet" patient waited, she slid to a stop and entered at a walk. I was struck by the fact that when this particular blood pressure machine was briskly walked, I could not hear it from the nursing station, but that when the nurse broke into a fast walk, the wheels on the blood pressure machine sounded like distant machine-gun fire.

As I was thinking about this sudden burst of speed, a nurse approached the desk, and said to the clerk: "Mr. X in 627 wants another pot of coffee." The clerk called the Dietary Department, and asked for Miss Y, exchanged a few pleasantries, and then asked for a second pot of coffee for Mr. X in room 627. Three minutes later a pot of coffee arrived on the dumbwaiter and was immediately takn into room 627.

It may reassure my readers to know that in this and other cases of "red carpet" conflict, the nurses were aware of their resentment at being ordered to provide "red carpet" treatment, but they were not aware that they were systematically sabotaging the excellent care that they were otherwise providing. In this particular case, the nurses were not aware that the noise of racing wheels bothered the patient. They were trying to tell him that they were very busy and that he was lucky to get first class care. They had forgotten his single reference to his feeling disoriented because from his window he could see only sky. One nurse immediately left our postmortem to put this matter right. They were not aware they had fallen into the trap of asking for extra coffee for this particular patient in a manner calculated to trigger a refusal from Dietary, but a similar request for Mr. X in room 627 had elicited an opposite response. They were aware that they were deliberately waking and washing the "red carpet" patient at six o'clock in the morning, but they had rationalized this behavior as necessary "because of the pressure of work."

The nurse provides care, and her first concern is, naturally enough, the needs of individual patients. It is difficult for her not to resent an order for "red carpet" treatment. This kind of order seems to suggest that she cannot be relied on to give each patient the best possible care. The nurse does not resent the "poor" patient merely because he cannot afford to pay for the care that he needs. The nurse does not take kindly to irresponsibility in any patient rich or poor: The "poor" patient who "refuses to learn" and the "rich" patient who "refuses to listen" are both frustating patients as far as the nurse is concerned.

The physician and the administrator are rarely in conflict over the affluent patient, but they sometimes come into conflict over a patient who cannot be expected to pay his bill. These conflicts occasionally become disputes about the right to decide whether or not a particular patient should be hospitalized. The right to decide when a sick person is to be hospitalized is firmly located within the physician's decision-making territories. The responsibility for keeping the hospital solvent belongs to the hospital administrator. This division of responsibility and authority breeds an interesting battle unless it is properly handled by both the administrator and the physician. The lay administrator and the physicians who use the hospital's facilities for their patients tend to border-fight about the decision to hospitalize those sick persons who cannot be expected to pay their bills. I will use the "pink-form" battle that was observed in one hospital to demonstrate the ritualized decision-making fights that characterize border-fights between hospital administrators and physicians. This particular "battle sequence" was observed a number of years ago by a colleague of mine, and for reasons that will become obvious, his name has been withheld.

> Every three or four months, a pile of pink forms began to accumulate on the right-hand side of the hospital director's desk. These pink forms were used by the local physicians to introduce a patient, whom the physician had arranged to hospitalize, to the hospital's Admission Office. The perspective patient presented the pink form; was interviewed, and in due course, admitted to the hospital bed. Under normal circumstances the pink form was then filed in a cabinet in the Admission Office.

The question was: Why were these pink forms piled on the director's desk rather than filed in the Admission Office; and what had happened to the patients to whom these pink forms referred? This is the story:

> Sometimes the Admission Office *questioned* the physician's decision to hospitalize a patient either because the patient owed the hospital money or because the patient was a poor financial risk. When this happened, the patient took the pink form back to his physician, and if the physician decided that his patient needed to be hospitalized whether or not he was a poor financial risk, the physician would write the word "Emergency" across the form, and send the patient back to the Admission Office. When the patient presented the pink form with "Emergency" written across it, he was admitted to a hospital bed, and the pink form was taken to the director's office.
>
> The interesting thing is that the pink forms with "Emergency" written across them do not crop up every now and then in a haphazard manner. In this particular hospital the pink-form phenomenon broke out at regular intervals: Every three or four months for a period of about ten days some patients were admitted as "Emergency" cases after an initial refusal. During a three-year period these border-fights broke out, on average, at three and one-half month intervals, and each incident lasted about ten days. The forms accumulated rather slowly at first, and reached a peak during the last three days of the battle. The word "Emergency" was small at first, and written in various colors. Toward the end of each conflict, the word "Emergency" expanded until it made the maximum use of available space. The bigger the word "Emergency" became, the more frequently it was written in red.

What happened behind the scenes, and why does this kind of border-fighting break out? Hospital administration does not challenge the physician's right to make an honest medical decision, but it does suspect that the physician is capable of exaggerating a sick person's needs in order to get him into a hospital bed. This suspicion is not always well founded: The physician recognizes a traditional responsibility to save expense for the low-income family whenever possible, and he realizes that the resources of the hospital are limited. The suspicion is present, however, and it periodically precipitates ritualized border-fights between hospital administration and the physicians.

The pink-form battle began before the first formal refusal was made, and I call the first phase of this battle the verbal phase.

> A person in the Admission Office voices a suspicion about a particular physician. This suspicion is supported by anecdotal information about the physician's extravagances on his patients' behalf. Other physicians are added to the list of "extravagant" physicians. The records of suspected cases are examined and the expert opinion of a person in Medical Records is sought.

The second phase of this battle, the cat and mouse phase, begins when each request for a hospital bed by any physician on the suspect list is carefully scrutinized.

> When a good refusal-opportunity comes along the Admission Office pounces. The prospective patient is refused admission, and is instructed to return to his physician. It is made quite clear to the patient that he *will be admitted* when he returns as a declared emergency. When the patient returns, he is admitted immediately, but the pink form with "Emergency" written on it is *not* filed in the Admission Office: It is *taken* to the director's office.

Once the battle breaks into the open, it tends to accelerate, and it is in its penultimate phase.

> The full resources of Medical Records are mobilized, and the cases against the offending physicians are documented. The battle usually ends in a noisy scene during which the physicians and the hospital director argue with each other. Sometimes the physicians initiate the final scene, and sometimes the director calls the physicians to account.

In either case, after the traditional shouting has died down, a new *modus vivendi* is reached, and the battle between the administrator and the physician is "cooled" for another quarter of a year.

Although the pink-form battle was fought more than fifteen years ago, the basic conflict between administrators and physicians has not been resolved. The administrator is accountable for hospital resources, and he periodically reminds the physician in one way or another of this. In a similar manner, physicians continue to remind administrators that their right to decide to use the hospital and its resources to the best interest of their patients must not be infringed. Consequently, ritualized border-fights about medical decisions which deplete hospital resources will persist. Although they may be less overt than the one described above, the way in which they are developed and resolved will be patterned in a similar manner: uneasiness about the physicians' use of hospital resources, collecting evidence to support the notion that they are being used recklessly, questioning specific decisions, confrontation, resolution, and temporary peace.

Similarly, the nurse's response to the ability of patients to pay for the care they need has not altered. Suggestions that special consideration be shown to wealthy and otherwise influential patients, however delicately phrased, inevitably are responded to as if they were attacks on the nurse's professional integrity. The wise administrator avoids appearing to request "red carpet" treatment, and the prudent patient makes it quite clear that he does not expect preferential treatment.

The nurse, the physician, and the administrator are not the only specialists with conflicting frames of reference: All categories of hospital specialists have their own unique frames of reference, and they all come into conflict with other categories of specialists. These conflicts are extremely interesting, and I am going to describe next how I use frame-of-reference conflicts to identify the decision-making territories of hospital specialists.

Ritualized fighting similar to the pink-form battle is a phenomenon that occurs over and over again in a society such as ours where knowledge changes rapidly, where new specialities emerge, and where the vested interests of old specialties shift. To the observer this kind of behavior is similar to the territorial behavior of other species, and I have come to think of the characteristic decision-making rights of any specialized group of people as if each unique combination of these rights is a separate territory, marked off by boundaries and defended by those to whom the right to make the decisions in it belongs.

Looked at from this point of view, the pink-form battle tells us something about the boundary that separates the administrator's decision-making territories from the physician's decision-making territories. The physician has the right to decide whether or not a sick person needs to be hospitalized, and the administrator has the right to make final decisions about how money is to be spent and collected. The administrator has a vested interest in the physician's decision to hospitalize his patient: If the patient can afford to pay his bill, it helps to keep the hospital out of debt. If the bill cannot be paid, the administrator must find some way to make up this deficit.

At first glance ritualized fighting about hospital admission suggests that administration is attempting to extend its decision-making boundaries by splitting the decision to hospitalize the patient into two parts: A diagnostic decision by the physician and a financial-feasibility decision by hospital administration. As far as this particular boundary dispute is concerned, other issues are at stake; and it would be unwise to leap to a quick conclusion. The central problem is funding. The hospital is a facility that the individual community needs but cannot afford. Traditional methods of funding the hospital are no longer adequate; and until a satisfactory solution to this problem is reached, hospital administrators will continue to *appear* to question the physician's right to hospitalize the patient who cannot pay his hospital bill.

When one examines the dynamics of the pink-form battle from this point of view, one begins to understand what is happening. Administration is reminding the physician that the hospital must remain solvent, and it is asking the physician for assurance that the financial situation of the patient and the hospital has been taken into consideration. The physician takes the patient's financial situation into consideration, but he does not routinely make this fact clear to the hospital.

The physician does consider ability to pay as well as diagnostic predicament before he decides to hospitalize a patient: He considers both the sick person's need for medical care and the sick person's ability to pay for what he needs. He also considers the added burden to the family of hospital bills. In most cases these calculations are not visible to the administrator who sometimes suspects that the physician is reckless with the limited resources of the hospital. When this suspicion is present, the hospital administrator is compelled to remind the physician that hospital resources are limited.

I once amused myself by translating the physician's recognition of both medical need and ability to pay into formulas that would make hospital administration less uneasy about the physician's willingness to recognize the economic needs of the hospital. With the help of a friendly physician, I drew up a hierarchy of diagnostic categories. Impending death, childbirth, insanity, and other conditions customarily institutionalized even when the patient's ability to pay is absolutely nil were at the top of the list as plus diagnoses $(+ D_x)$. Minor complaints, for example, an operation for one ingrown toenail, were at the bottom of the list as minus diagnoses $(- D_x)$. The patient's ability to pay was ranked with plus and minus dollar signs. This approach yielded the following formulas:

$$(+ D_x) + (+ \$) \qquad = \text{hospital sickness}$$
$$(+ D_x) + (- \$) \qquad = \text{hospital sickness}$$
$$(- D_x) + (+ \$) \qquad = \text{hospital sickness}$$
$$(- D_x) + (- \$) \text{ does } not - \text{hospital sickness}$$

The physician routinely uses this formula *before* he decides to hospitalize a patient. He realizes that hospital sickness, being sick enough to qualify for hospital admission, is not always defined by diagnostic categories. The administrator and the physician both know that the poorer you are, the sicker you must be in order to become a hospital patient; but the administrator sometimes wonders whether the physician has forgotten this. It seems to me that if the physician would add a hospital sickness formula to his requests for admission, the administrator's suspicion that he is reckless with hospital resources might decrease.

In cases in which established decision-making boundaries are not complicated by other factors, ritual fights may be used to remind those concerned about exactly where the boundary lines are drawn. In these cases the most recently established speciality tends to take the initiative. A case in point is the way in which the radiologist reminds the physician that the right to make two decisions no longer belongs to the physician. The final decision about how patients are to be prepared for x-ray examination, and the decision to stop exposing a patient to x-ray, initially medical decisions, now are located in the radiologist's decision-making territory.

It sometimes seems to the physician that the radiologist makes arbitrary decisions when he refuses to subject individual patients to further x-ray exposure. A number of physicians have expressed it as their opinion that radiologists use these refusals to remind physicians that *they* know more about this matter than physicians do: As one internist said: "This is their way of showing us who is boss." It seems reasonable to assume that some x-ray refusals are boundary markers.

The fact that arbitrary action about preparing patients for x-ray procedures is boundary-fighting can be documented by more than mere opinion. For example, there are a number of acceptable ways in which a patient can be prepared for a barium enema, but most x-ray departments insist that all patients must be prepared for this procedure in one way, and the particular way selected varies from x-ray department to x-ray department. Occasionally, a physician asks the radiologist to give a barium enema to a patient who has been or will be prepared for this procedure in an alternate, but medically acceptable, manner. Most frequently, the radiologist refuses. In some cases the physician is trying to pick a fight; in most cases, however, the physician's request is reasonable and, in his opinion, to the best interests of his patient: Under these circumstances, I consider the radiologist's refusal to be boundary-fighting. This state of affairs sometimes becomes visible when a new head of radiology is appointed. The routine preparation for a barium enema frequently changes with a change in leadership. I have sometimes wondered whether radiologists use a change of this type to put their individual stamp on a department.

The radiologist has specialized a territory that originally belonged to the physician, and he tends to take the initiative in reminding the physician that radiologists now make decisions about x-ray procedures. This ritualized boundary-marking characterizes new specialities that have been carved out of older specialities. As far as the radiologist is concerned his boundary-marking behavior is a dialogue with the physician, and it does not include arguments with other categories of hospital specialists.

When the new speciality has been carved out of territory that did not previously belong exclusively to the physician, boundary-marking behavior tends to become complex. Some of the functions that have been delegated by the nurse are excellent examples. At one time final decisions about housekeeping and the diet kitchen were located in the nurse's decision-making territory. These functions have been delegated to dietitians and to housekeepers, and the nurse now requests services from these departments. She no longer makes decisions about how these services should be rendered. In these two cases boundary-marking behavior is complicated by the physician's traditional right to make decisions about cleanliness and about diet. That the physician has, and continues to exercise, these traditional decision-making rights makes it necessary for the dietitian and the housekeeper to mark two sets of boundaries: one with the nurse and one with the physician.

The dietitian is a diet expert, and the physician's right to make decisions about what his patient should eat challenges the dietitian's specialized knowledge. The dietitian's behavior suggests an attempt to establish the right to make decisions about modality. The therapeutic dietitian sometimes acts as if honor could be satisfied if the physician would name the disease, and then permit the dietitian to decide which particular diet would be most therapeutic. Two characteristic behavior patterns support this impression: dietary handbook behavior and demonstrations about the relationship between food and the human body.

Many dietary departments prepare a handbook in which a collection of different therapeutic diets are described and numbered. The physicians are asked to order by number out of this book. Many physicians find this approach cumbersome, and continue to order by simple description, salt-free diet, for example, without making other possible specifications. There were a number of salt-free diets in the handbook I examined. It was explained to me that when the physician wrote salt-free diet, he usually wanted a normal diet without salt. There were other possible variations, however, and it was explained to me that the dietary department had a responsibility to make absolutely certain that the physician knew what he was ordering. Until his order was sufficiently specific, the food tray was withheld. Most of the physicians did not recognize this behavior as boundary-fighting. It was seen by them as irritating behavior that sometimes inconvenienced their patients.

The other characteristic attempt at boundary-fighting is rarely observed by the physician although medical students sometimes are invited to attend the demonstrations. These skirmishes do not inconvenience the patient. They are intended to show how little physicians know about the relationship between food and the human body. They also express the dietary department's suspicion that nurses and physician sometimes eat the food they order for their patients. The most striking example that I have observed with a demonstration and lecture. During the demonstration a sirloin steak was placed on a platter, and a bottle of coke was poured into the depressed center of it. The steak was locked into a closet and the key to the closet was placed in the safekeeping of a member of the audience. Twenty-four hours later the audience reassembled, the closet was opened, and the steak was examined. The hollow into which the coke had been poured had become tender, and it now was possible to work a finger through the meat.

The audience was given statistical information about the numbers of cokes and other soft drinks ordered for the patients on each of the surgical units. They were asked to think about what was happening to the stomach linings of the patients on the surgical units. After a brief pause a reassuring note was struck: the plight of the patients on the surgical units was not as bad as it seemed, apparently the staff on those units drank most of the soft drinks that were ordered for the patients.

This particular demonstration was repeated every four or five months, and it was well attended. It was dramatic, but it did not convey the message intended. The audience knew that live tissue did not behave like dead meat, and they knew that under normal circumstances coke does not stay in the human stomach long enough to marinate it. This particular dietitian had overplayed her hand, but her attempt to establish a reputation for superior knowledge in this area was not otherwise uncharacteristic.

This particular phenomenon most frequently manifests itself in a less dramatic manner, and the following extracts from my field diary are typical:

> Dietitian to housekeeper: "Seven cases of coke in one week. Either those surgeons don't know what coke does to their patients or they are drinking it themselves."

> Dietitian to observer: "Dr. Y always orders a tray for his patients while they are in the delivery suite. His excuse is that when they have delivered, the kitchen will be closed. I looked it up: patients shouldn't eat before delivery, and in most cases they're in no shape to eat after it. Obviously, Dr. Y orders a tray because *he* wants to eat."

> Dietitian to Medical Records librarian: "You're not the only one with a problem about pediatrics. Nurse S had a conference to tell me that her patients like bananas and they like peanut butter, but they won't eat "bananas with peanut butter smeared on them." I know who put *that* idea into their heads: when Nurse D was in charge the kids ate those salads and liked them."

> Dietitian to observer: "Every year it's the same. It takes three months to teach the new residents how to order diets. They may have got away with writing out what they think they want in the hospitals they came from, but that's not good enough here: We're a teaching hospital."

The dietitian, the housekeeper, the Medical Records librarian and the heads of other service departments tend to complain to each other about the behavior of physicians and nurses. Frequently, one or two nurses in supervisory positions are made members of this complaining circle. The department heads describe these nurses as "What good nurses used to be like."

Boundary-fights with nurses are particularly interesting. The nurse's decision-making rights are not clear-cut. Many functions previously performed by the nurse have been either delegated to or preempted by others.

New functions have appeared, and some of these functions impinge on nursing functions. In addition, the nurse's decision-making territories expand and contract to accommodate institutional slack. As a consequence, the nursing profession finds it difficult to define the nurse's function, and the nurse is not absolutely sure what is included in and excluded from her decision-making territories.

The nurse's fluctuating decision-making patterns are most visible in the hospital setting in which the needs of the patient must be met during an entire twenty-four-hour day and for a seven-day week. Other services and the hospital's facilities are manned for a shorter work week, in some cases as short as forty hours. This arrangement creates problems that can be solved only when the nurse mobilizes nonnursing activities to meet those patient needs that cannot wait until hibernating services are reactivated. Drugs, food, and other facilities are sometimes needed when those who normally supply them are not on the premises. The patients' urgent needs sometimes force the nurse to assume alien functions. This periodic need to function in alien territories gives the nurse a sense of vested interest that complicates her decision-making battles.

It is obvious that moving in and out of different territories must make it difficult for the nurse to identify her unique decision-making rights. Consequently, she is not sure what rights she should defend; and it may well be that when she attempts to defend her territory, her ability to do so vigorously has been eroded. The nurse's apparent confusion about boundaries characteristically is expressed as doubts and regrets. The following excerpts from my field diary are examples:

> We never should have let Dietary take over food.

> Should we let the doctors fight administration for more nursing staff or is this (fight) our business?

> The way in which patients are transported from one part of the hospital to another is most unsatisfactory. The question is: Does nursing have the right to do anything about it?

Comments such as these suggest not only that the nurse's decision-making territory is not clearly defined but also that the patient may suffer the consequence.

Another interesting phenomenon is the latent decision-making right, and what I call the "recreation skirmish" is an excellent example of what happens when a latent right to make decisions is questioned. It is now customary to provide recreation for hospitalized children and for psychiatric patients. The nurse and the occupational therapist both have a vested interest in recreation. The nurse has traditionally provided some sort of recreational facilities for these patients, and she continues to do something about recreation during the evenings and weekends. Occupational therapists are of two minds about recreation. They know that recreation is a therapeutic vehicle, and that if it is acknowledged by others as such, they are prepared to give it a home until it develops into a full-fledged discipline. Although occupational therapists operate on the proverbial shoestring, they are extremely resourceful. Consequently, they stake a claim to recreation if, and when, the issue is raised. The nurse and the physician usually are unaware that recreation is a therapeutic vehicle, and they tend to stir up unintended skirmishes by suggesting that: "someone be brought in to do something about the patients' spare time."

Why should such a seemingly harmless suggestion stir up a border-fight? As far as the physician and the nurse are concerned, the patients' spare time rarely has had more than nuisance value, and their recreation offerings have been, for the most part, mere attempts to keep the idle patient out of mischief. The occupational therapist, on the other hand, has used the patients' idle hands to create a most interesting therapeutic approach. They use everyday materials in a culture that sets store by complicated machinery. And they use these materials to mobilize the patient as a person. If he is physically handicapped, they teach him to eat, to dress himself, and to fry eggs as expertly as the "normal" person is able to do these things. If he is damaged in less visible ways, they help him to build social competence by encouraging creative relationships with paper, paint, clay, metals, leather, and other ordinary materials. Much of what they do with patients looks like play, but they use a label that reminds us of the value that our society sets on productiveness. Occupational therapists provide hours of excellent therapy for mere cents per patient day, but the apparent frivolity of their therapeutic tools makes them hesitant to ask for adequate financial support and they operate in a resourceful manner on a shoestring.

As far as the occupational therapist is concerned, recreation is a fallow territory. As long as the issue is not raised, the recreation of the patients will be allowed to limp on. The occupational therapist will do as much as time and other resources permit, and she will be delighted when the nurse and the physician add to the patients' recreational diet. But when either the nurse or the physician suggests that a lay person with no therapeutic training might be brought in to "do something about the patients' spare time," the occupational therapist is honor-bound to act. This action comes as a surprise to the nurse and to the physician. As one pediatric nurse expressed it: "I did not realize that anyone thought they owned our playroom."

Recreational skirmishes are interesting. Until recreational therapy is well established as a separate discipline, any attempt to formalize recreation forces the occupational therapist to lay claim to the decision-making rights involved even though the department may not have the resources to assume the additional responsibility. This claim to recreation draws attention to the fact that occupational therapy has developed against the grain of a Puritan value system, and explains why this discipline continues to operate on a shoestring despite its productiveness. That the nurse and the physician are unaware of the occupational therapist's claim to recreation merely confirms the preceding statements. Recreation is an excellent example of a latent decision-making territory.

Although I had studied a number of other segments of contemporary western society, I did not become aware of the full significance of the decision-making boundaries that separate one specialized group of people from another specialized group of people until I began to study the hospital culture. In this particular setting, these boundaries are tremendously important, and it seems to me that all categories of hospital specialists might find it profitable to look at their chronic conflicts from this point of view. Chronic conflicts between groups of differently specialized people usually mean that the right to make specific decisions is in question. In most cases these conflicts will continue until the boundary between the two decision-making territories is clearly defined.

3

The Changing Hospital

In the first chapter I touched briefly on the changing shape of the hospital. In this chapter I intend to look more closely at one of the most recent changes in hospital behavior: the big business look. Most people do not think of the hospital as a big business, but hospitals are now referred to as one of the biggest industries in the country, and this classification is having an interesting effect on hospital behavior.

When hospitals think of themselves as part of an industry, they begin to adopt practices that have proved to be productive in industry. I call these innovations "big-business behavior." One of the interesting things about the hospital's big-business behavior is that much of it is used in a somewhat magical manner. The hospital tends to take over practices that have proved useful to industry without modifying these practices to fit a somewhat different set of conditions. The hospital makes the same *gestures* that industry makes, and it seems to expect the same results. The way in which many hospitals use costing-behavior is an excellent example. Costing-behavior has been extremely useful to industry. It has enabled industry to analyze its production costs, and to detect waste in its production systems. When these wasteful practices are corrected, industry is able to produce its product at a lower cost. The usefulness of costing-behavior is entirely dependent on the ability to produce accurate cost-figures. The accounting system that enables industry to produce such a figure is a cost-accounting system.

Most hospitals imitate industry's costing-behavior, but in many cases they have *not* adopted the kind of accounting system that will enable them to produce accurate cost-figures. Hospitals traditionally use a fund-accounting system, and many hospitals still use this system.[1] In these hospitals only two changes have been made. A complex system of inter-dependent funds has been accumulated. And a number of sophisticated machines have been imported to keep the monies in these funds in order. A fund-accounting system, however complex, is like a bank statement supplemented by check stubs and deposit slips: It tells you what came into the account and what went out of it. But it does not produce accurate cost-figures about every part of the operation. When hospitals with fund-accounting systems publish cost-figures it seems as if they imagine that they will automatically operate in a more economical manner by *acting* as if they were analyzing their production costs.

Hospitals exchange costing information with each other, and they seem to compete with each other to produce the lowest cost per whatever-it-is. Let me describe a case in point. Some years ago one hospital published a cost-per-meal figure. This figure was not accompanied by a statement about what had been included and excluded to arrive at the cost-figure, and there was no way of knowing whether or not the figures used in the original arithmetic were accurate cost-figures.

A competing hospital decided to reckon out its cost-per-meal, and this hospital's arithmetic was as follows:

I. Number of meals provided was figured as:
   a. number of patients plus number of staff (for number of mouths fed);
   b. the total number of people was multiplied by three (for three meals a day);
   c. and this figure was multiplied by 365 (for days in the year).

There were four obvious exaggerations. The staff were on a three-shift system. On one of the three shifts, the graveyard shift, no meal was served. No staff member ate more than one cafeteria meal in one day. Staff members worked 235, rather than 365, days a year.

II. Total cost of meals was assumed to be:
   a. wages of dietary staff;

[1] T. L. Martin, *Hospital Accounting: Principles and Practice,* 2d ed. (Chicago: Physicians Record Co., 1952).

    b. plus salaries of dietitians;

    c. plus cost of raw materials.

In this case the understatement was less obvious. No allowances had been made for overhead, depreciation or expendibles.

When the understated cost of meals was divided by the exaggerated number of meals, the resultant cost-figure was unsatisfactory from a competitive point of view. In order to remedy this fault, the salaries of the dietitians were removed from the cost-of-meals formula, and the resultant cost-per-meal was considered satisfactory. The rationale for this removal was that the dietitians had a teaching function as well as a food-management function. The mathematicians in this particular institution felt that the salaries of the dietitians could legitimately be excluded from meal costs, and no one concerned seemed to think that the rules of the game had been violated when the new, and lower, cost-figure was entered in competition with cost-figures from other hospitals without any statement about how it had been calculated.[2]

Hospitals sometimes use cost-figures to counter requests for salary increases. The classical example is to counter the request for an increase in nurses' salaries with nursing cost-figures. This move is effective because it mobilizes the nurses' sense of guilt, but the cost-figure used is not always accurate. In many hospitals the supposed cost of nursing is inflated, and there are two usual ways in which this is done. One inflation system adds the cost of all supplies and, in some cases, services used by the patient-care units to its nursing cost-figure. The other inflation system uses the percentage of staff approach. If 75 percent of the people employed by the hospital are Nursing Service personnel, then 75 percent of the cost of running the hospital is the amount that nursing is supposed to cost. It is obvious that neither system produces a valid cost-figure. And it may be useful to nurses to know that cost-figures can, and should be, questioned, even though some hospitals do use cost-accounting systems, and are capable of producing accurate cost-figures.

This particular example of "making business gestures" is beginning to disappear. It was encouraged by the way in which insurance companies pay hospital bills, and it is being discouraged by the way in which the federal government is paying for Medicare. It is usual practice for insurance companies to pay stated portions of specified charges, and in some cases generously enough to compensate partly for services that either will not be paid for or are inadequately paid for. Hospital billing practices have been patterned by the insurance company's paying practices, and as

---

[2] This example of costing-behavior was supplied by an informant who had been a consultant to this particular Dietary Department at the time it was "manufacturing" its cost-per-meal figure.

one hospital administrator remarked, "There's no percentage in producing accurate cost-figures." The federal government has approached the payment of hospital bills in a different manner. It pays in relation to stated costs of itemized services rendered; and although many hospitals are unable to make more than estimates of the actual cost of itemized services, the necessity of preparing this kind of bill and the fact that items on it may be, and sometimes are, queried is encouraging hospitals to adopt cost-accounting systems. There now is a "percentage in producing accurate cost-figures." Nevertheless, business gesturing is increasing rather than decreasing, and an examination of it has led me to suspect an interesting possibility.

At the present time the systems-engineering game seems to be displacing the cost-figure game. At first glance what the systems engineer is doing in the hospital does not seem to be a game. He can be seen using sophisticated techniques, and in some cases complex equipment, as he examines and analyzes existing processes and procedures; he is serious and conscientious; and his reports make impressive statements that seem to show how the hospital can function in a more efficient manner. However, as a number of systems engineers have explained to me, most of these studies, although valid, are not producing information that can be used by hospital workers. This is particularly true of the primary function of the hospital: diagnosing, treating, and caring for patients. In short, the systems engineer has produced analyses that can be implemented about such things as assembling food trays, but although he can analyze patient-care in a manner satisfactory to himself, the results frequently give meaningless information as far as physicians, nurses, and other hospital specialists are concerned. Eventually, the systems engineering game will become more than a game, and I suspect that it will do so when physicians, nurses, and other health practitioners begin to use the techniques developed by systems engineers to examine what they do and how they do it.

The question that interested me was: Why does apparently unproductive behavior of this kind continue year after year until it either becomes unfashionable to use a particular gesture or a particular gesture accidentally becomes productive? When I question hospital administrators about this phenomenon, they usually begin by defending the rationale for spending money in this way, and end by saying such things as: "It looks good." "It might pay off." "So and so (on the board) is a 'nut' about these things." These responses caused me to speculate about the management of organizations that are not expected to make money: prisons, schools, hospitals, cities, government departments, and so forth. As far as hospitals are concerned, their administrators move to superior positions by going from one hospital to another or from smaller to larger hospitals.

These moves are relatively rapid, and other categories of hospital specialists comment on them by saying: "We get a new batch of bright young men in that office every two or three years." An examination of the relationship between the demand for hospital administrators and the supply of those persons with Masters degrees in Hospital Administration suggests that supply and demand might be one passport to promotion.[3] One hospital administrator who was unusually frank while discussing this possibility said: "So, why sweat it? Supply and demand will see to it that on my fourth move I will be in charge of a hospital with 1,000 employees under me." According to my observations, most hospital administrators do not act as if this is their attitude. They spend a great deal of time on the job, and they seem to take the hospital's problems seriously. But they do change jobs more frequently than other top-ranking hospital specialists.

During the past years, hospitals have consciously increased their big-business behavior, and we can expect such behavior to continue increasing. Another, less obvious and more important, imitation of industry, a change from centralized to decentralized management, has begun. This change should be understood by those who work in hospitals because it provides them with a unique opportunity to eliminate some of the problems that were created when patient-care was institutionalized. We will examine this important change in considerable detail in another chapter. In the present chapter, we will place this significant change in historical context.

For some years a quiet revolution in the organizational style of large-scale institutions has been in progress. This revolution has been quiet because the changes that have been made are not widely recognized as significant. Although they do not clearly understand what is happening to them, our large-scale institutions are changing from one organizational system to another: They are changing from a bureaucratic form of organization to a corporate form of organization. This change is significant because it reverses a decision that was made over a century ago. In order to understand what is happening to our large-scale institutions, including our hospitals, it is necessary to go back to the beginning of the Industrial Revolution, and to reexamine the way in which men and machines originally were organized into production teams.

In 1938, when I was studying with Mauss[4] at the College de France in Paris, I came across some documents that are pertinent to our understanding of the social problems that were built into the way in which

---

[3] Florio makes a similar point about city managers. G. K. Florio, "Continuity in City-Manager Careers," *Amer. J. Sociol.* 62 (1956): 253–263.

[4] Mauss was a French sociologist who is thought of as one of the "European theorists," and is probably best known in this country for *The Gift*. Marcel Mauss, *The Gift*, I. Cunnison, trans. (New York: The Free Press, 1954).

western societies organized men and machines into production teams. These documents were handwritten records of a series of discussions that took place between social theorists at the Sorbonne. My notes about these documents were destroyed during World War II, but my memory of the argument presented is vivid enough to make notes unnecessary. To the best of my recollection, these discussions took place in the late 1830s. At that time the intellectual climate in Paris would have been ripe for discussions of this type. Comte [5] manufactured the label "sociology" in 1822, and his notion that the primary function of sociology was to recreate society by engineering social change was being taken quite seriously by European intellectuals during the second quarter of the nineteenth century.

This document recorded a discussion about how men and machines were to be organized together to produce goods. One side argued that the machine should set the style and pace of the production line. It seemed sensible to the scholars on this side of the argument that all the work on the production line should be divided into machine-sized tasks. It was obvious that machines with new capabilities would be invented. And they argued that if the production line was designed for machines, people could be replaced by machines without rearranging the way in which the production line was organized. The scholars on the other side of the argument agreed with this logic, but they contended that humans would not and could not adapt to a working situation which deprived them of a sense of self-determination and a sense of working cooperatively with others.

Both sides agreed that it would be most practical to give the worker a job fit for a machine, and the part-time role of a submachine. [6] One side doubted man's ability to function in this manner. Those in favor of the submachine role countered this doubt by arguing that the "workers" would be drawn from the "lower classes." It seemed to these scholars that "lower class" man set his highest value on material goods. They agreed that it would be difficult for the "worker" to play the submachine role, but they felt that he would be prepared to do so if his material level was raised, and if his working day was shortened. The discussion recorded in the document I examined was merely one of many such discussions in

[5] Auguste Comte (1798–1857), French philosopher, sociologist, and founder of positivism.

[6] This label was suggested by the work of Gulick and Fayol whose writings about the division of labor in organizations seemed to view the employee either as an appendage to an incomplete machine or as an "inert instrument." H. Fayol, *Industrial and General Administration* (London: Sir Isaac Pitman & Sons, Ltd., 1930). L. Gulick and L. Urwick, eds. *Papers on the Science of Administration* (New York: Institute of Public Administration, 1937), p. 3.

France and in other European countries, that set the stage for the way in which western societies eventually decided to organize men and machines into teams to produce goods.

When I read this document in 1938, I did not realize that I was judging its contents out of historical context. In the 1830s, the material level in Europe was extremely low: One could be hanged for stealing a sheep. In those days the argument that a "lower class" man who risked his life to steal a sheep placed his highest value on material goods would have seemed valid. The record of this discussion aroused my interest in the mass-production factory. I became curious about the institution that seemed to have successfully imposed the submachine role.

The mass-production factory that I studied for two and one-half years was organized in a bureaucratic manner, it characteristically centralized decision-making, and it used a rationalized pay system. The production workers in this particular factory responded to the organizational style of the institution and to its rationalized pay system in a characteristic manner. They organized themselves into an informal system that increased their sense of working cooperatively with others. And at a critical point in the formal system, informal action was taken to prevent the formal system from imposing what the workers considered an unfair decision about pay.

A great deal has been written about a bureaucratic system of organization that characteristically produces an informal system so vigorous that if the two systems, formal and informal, do not have compatible objectives, the formal system cannot achieve its objectives.[7] Those who are acquainted with the behavior of large-scale organizations will have encountered numerous examples of this phenomenon. Some theorists have gone so far as to conclude that a bureaucratic system could not function if it were not assisted by the informal system. This particular notion was tested on a grand scale some years ago when the English postal system, unable to strike in the usual manner because its workers were government employees, abandoned their informal system, and insisted on functioning according to formal rules and regulations. Everyone worked as long and as hard as usual, but all post office employees were meticulous about doing everything through formal channels and according to officially prescribed procedures. Within two weeks the system was unable to accept mail. There was no more space in post office buildings, and it was reported in the press that it was no longer possible to insert postcards into English mailboxes. This interesting strike supports the contention that a bureaucratic system cannot function without assistance from the informal system and it introduced the notion of striking "by the book," as strikes of this kind have come to be called.

[7] For a more explicit model, *see* T. Parsons, *Structure and Process in Modern Society* (New York: The Free Press, 1960).

Why should an elegantly logical system of organization break down in this astonishing manner? A bureaucratic form of organization is rational, and it is designed to protect the operation of the institution from the vagaries of people. Max Weber,[8] a classical guide to the bureaucratic form of organization, saw such a system as the most efficient instrument for the accomplishment of large-scale tasks. From a theoretical point of view, this is true. In practice, however, the system does tend to become nonfunctional.

It becomes nonfunctional because of the tug-of-war between people and the system. Those who man a bureaucratic system seem to insist on working cooperatively with each other, and they refuse to let the system impose on them. The system responds by accumulating red tape, and in a relatively short period of time, it cannot function unless these accumulations are by-passed. A state of affairs that could be corrected if periodic red-tape pruning were to become routine practice.

This phenomenon can best be understood when we look at the decision-making patterns that characterize bureaucratic systems.[9] Let us pretend that the bureaucratic pyramid is drawn in people rather than offices, and let us block in the heads of the people in that system to show how the bureaucracy's insistence on centralizing decision-making deprives most of those who work in this system of a sense of self-determination and of the opportunity to work cooperatively with others. When this has been done, I think that you will understand why humans characteristically respond to a bureaucratic system by developing a strong and vigorous informal system of organization and behavior. A bureaucratic system drawn as people rather than as offices would look something like that shown in Figure 4.

In a bureaucratic system, decision-making is centralized toward the head of the top person in the pyramid. This top head makes decisions about what those immediately below him in the system will do; and these heads, in turn, make decisions about the actions of those immediately below them. At each descending level the opportunity to make decisions decreases. At the lowest level in this type of system, people are expected to do what they have been told to do as they are told to do it. At the lowest level in the bureaucratic pyramid, people have the right to make one decision: the decision to quit. Cooperative action about decisions made at higher levels in the hierarchy are a threat to this decision-making system. Problems that could be solved by cooperative action at functional levels are

[8] Max Weber, a sociologist, is one of the two primary shapers of theory about organization. For a fuller statement, see the notes at the end of this book.

[9] C. I. Barnard, the other primary shaper of our theories about organization, concluded that decision-making is the essence of formal organization. C. I. Barnard, *The Function of the Executive* (Cambridge, Mass.: Harvard University Press, 1938).

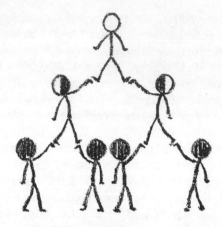

Figure 4.

supposed to be formally resolved at an appropriate superior level. This correct bureaucratic behavior is called "going through channels."

The human apparently finds it extremely difficult to function according to this depersonalized logic, and a bureaucratic system characteristically produces informal action and an informal system based on man's insistence on retaining some sense of self-determination (Parsons 1960). This insistence violates the system in two ways. Those at middle levels by-pass correct communication channels in order to work cooperatively with each other. And those at lower levels in the hierarchy cooperate to prevent the system from imposing what they consider unreasonable decisions. The system responds by accumulating red tape.

The bureaucratic system's red-tape accumulating patterns are interesting. Lower-level resistence causes procedures to break down at functional levels. The system characteristically responds by introducing additional procedures designed to prevent the initial break. Continued resistance produces a new break either in another part of the operation or in the new procedures. In either case the system produces another set of remedial procedures, and in this manner accumulates cumbersome procedures that are not functional unless they are short-circuited by informal action. The middle-level practice of by-passing correct communication channels permits red tape to accumulate in a somewhat different manner. The correct procedures that are passed down from higher levels are not put to the test, and the flaws in these procedures are not detected and corrected. If informal action at the middle level is effective, which it frequently is, those at higher levels tend to assume that the system is functioning productively because *their* directives had exceptional merit. This assumption encourages them to produce additional red tape.

When sufficient red tape has been accumulated, the formal system's ability to function effectively inevitably becomes dependent on the compatability of the informal system's objectives. When the formal system and the informal system have common or compatible objectives, a bureaucracy is functional; but when their objectives are opposed, a bureaucracy ceases to be functional. Anyone who has ever had anything to do with hospitals will know that hospitals are no exception to this rule. In a hospital the informal system always can, and sometimes does, defeat the formal system.

The tug-of-war between people and the system takes place at all but the highest levels in the bureaucratic pyramid. At the lowest levels it produces a phenomenon that is gradually changing the organizational form of the large-scale institutions in our society. In a bureaucratic system the lowest level of management and the highest level of worker or inmate take informal, cooperative action to prevent the formal system from making excessive demands on those who occupy positions at lower levels in the formal system. This protective action is so strong that it can be changed, but it cannot be broken. The characteristic response of those at lower levels in the hierarchy to the depersonalized logic of the bureaucratic system has created sufficient pressure to change the organizational style of large-scale institutions. This interesting phenomenon is not always clearly understood, and I will describe two examples: one in a mental hospital, and the other in a mass-production factory.

Belknap [10] published a significant study about a mental hospital ward. In this study he describes how the attendants (lowest level of supervision) and the trusties (highest level of patient) cooperated to impose a reward and punishment system that enabled the attendants to control the patient-population. In the ward in which Belknap studied, shock therapy was part of this reward and punishment system. That Belknap was able to prove that the attendants rather than the physicians decided which patients would receive shock therapy is so startling that the significance of the phenomenon Belknap described is not always recognized. Belknap is saying that when the formal system makes impossible demands on the lowest level of staff, those at this level collaborated with those immediately below them in the institution's hierarchy to prevent the system from making an impossible demand.

In this case the system expected too few attendants to control too many patients, and it expected them to do so in a therapeutic manner. This expectation was an impossible demand. The attendants reduced an impossible demand to what they considered a possible demand by cooperating with the trusties to impose a reward and punishment system that would effectively control the patient-population. This is the classical solution to the problem that is created when too few people are expected to control too many people.

[10] I. Belknap, *Human Problems of a State Hospital* (New York: McGraw-Hill, Inc., Blakiston Division, 1956).

The attendants were able to incorporate shock therapy into their reward and punishment system by making opportunistic use of the fact that the nurses and the physicians were not numerous enough to observe patient behavior. The decision to use shock therapy is based on certain changes in the patient's behavior. In this particular hospital the physicians were dependent on the nurses for information about changes in patient behavior, and the nurses based their reports to the physicians on information supplied to them by the attendants. The attendants were in a strategic position to impose shock therapy as a punishment, and they made use of this opportunity.

In 1940, in a mass-production factory in England, I encountered what I now call the Belknap phenomenon. The pay system in this particular factory worked in the following manner. A rate was set on each job, and this rate permitted the average worker to earn time and one-third. If any worker consistently earned more than time and one-half on any job, that job was retimed, and a lower rate was set. When the production system broke down, the worker was deprived of the opportunity to work, and he was placed on waiting time. When he was on waiting time, the worker was paid his basic rate. If his basic rate was $1 an hour, a worker was in danger of being fired unless he produced enough to earn $1.33 an hour. He was in danger of having the rate changed if he showed himself able to earn more than $1.50 an hour, a change that would adversely affect others on the same job. And he was arbitrarily paid $1 an hour when, through no fault of his own, the system broke down, and he was unable to work. Pay systems similar to the one described above were used at that time in most factories, and the "banking system" that I am about to describe was a characteristic response to this pay system.

From management's point of view, the firm was being extremely generous by paying the workers when they were not working. At that time, seasonal agricultural workers, for example, were not paid when the weather prevented them from working during parts of the workday. From the factory workers' point of view, however, the firm was penalizing them when *its* system broke down. Under these circumstances the workers recruited the lowest level of supervision (the charge hands), and cooperated with them to establish a "banking system" that wiped out what the workers felt was an injustice.

The banking system functioned in the following manner: All workers routinely produced more than enough to earn either time and one-third or time and one-half. All workers routinely checked their production in at a steady rate, no lower than time and one-third and no higher than time and one-half. Surplus production was routinely "banked" with the charge hand. The charge hand set this surplus to one side, and it was routinely drawn out of the charge hands "bank," and turned in to the "checker" as work done during waiting periods when the system had broken down. If the system did not break down sufficiently frequently, workers accumulated an embarrassing amount of surplus production in the "bank." Individuals in this predicament took unofficial holidays. During these holidays the charge hand would "clock" the absent worker in and out of the factory, and he would turn in a usual day's production for the absent worker. Such banking behavior was quite open, occurred in all factories that used a rationalized pay system, and was impossible to break. This banking system is an excellent example of the Belknap phenomenon.

The Belknap phenomenon enables those at lower levels in a bureaucratic system to modify the decisions made at higher levels in the hierarchy. As we shall see in the next chapter, the Belknap phenomenon tends to disappear as the institution decentralizes its decision-making to functional levels. When the decision-making process is decentralized, those at all levels in the system are given a voice in the decisions that directly affect their own working situations. Humans seem to function best when they retain some sense of controlling their own actions, and decentralized decision-making provides them with this sense. Unfortunately, this particular change in organizational style is not always clearly understood. This lack of understanding tends to be expressed in two ways: as mere democratic gesturing, and by allowing individuals to make decisions for which they cannot be held accountable. Empty gesturing is self-defeating, and allowing people to make inappropriate decisions produces chaos.

4

Decision-Making Patterns

In this chapter I am going to describe the way in which large-scale institutions, including hospitals, seem to be changing their decision-making patterns. Early in the Industrial Revolution, a bureaucratic system organized around centralized decision-making became the preferred model for institutions that produced goods, and this form of organization was gradually adopted by other large-scale institutions. People-processing plants took longer to convert to centralized decision-making than those institutions that produced other services. In this country, the last kind of people-processing plant to adopt centralized decision-making was the city public school system.[1]

During the past twenty years, the very period during which city public school systems were converting to centralized decision-making, an interesting change in the organizational style of large-scale institutions has become increasingly obvious: a change to decentralized decision-making. This

[1] For an extensive discussion of this process, *see* S. T. Kimball and J. E. Maclillan, Jr., *Education for the New America* (New York: Random House, Inc., 1962).

change is significant because it is a change from a bureaucratic form of administration to a corporate form of administration. This change, when it is completed, will have reversed the decision that was made at the beginning of the Industrial Revolution about how men and machines were to be organized into production teams.

The way in which this significant change is being made is interesting. Industry did not say to itself one day: "Let us abandon our bureaucratic form of administration by decentralizing our decision-making patterns." Industry began to change its organizational style by finding solutions to chronic problems. The "banking system" described in the last chapter was one of these problems.

During the period when I was studying industry, the science of man-management was in its infancy despite the fact that it had been over one hundred years since Auguste Comte had postulated that the primary function of sociology was to engineer social change. In the 1940s one of the problems that man-management specialists had recognized, and were attempting to solve, was a lack of morale and motivation at lower levels in the bureaucratic pyramid. At that time these specialists offered as solutions such schemes as suggestion boxes, birthday greetings from the firm, anual outings, piped in music, and lectures about how each worker's minute and repetitious task made an important contribution to the "product." They had identified the cause of the problem that they were trying to solve, lack of a sense of being part of the system, but they were mistaken about how to cure the disease. Their schemes were attempts to increase the workers' sense of social cohesion, but they did not seem to realize that humans need a sense of self-determination and a sense of working cooperatively with others in order to feel that they are part of a social system. When these basic human needs are not met, people tend to feel that they are being used by the institution for its own purposes.

The innovations primarily responsible for the unplanned, and in some cases undetected, decentralization of decision-making in industry was a new approach to this particular problem. Large-scale organizations find it extremely difficult to remain cohesive enough to function effectively, and a considerable expenditure of money and time is devoted to attempts at manufacturing social cohesion. Trading under different labels, the notion of giving the workers a "voice" in the various ways in which the institution organizes itself to function was the innovation primarily responsible for the quiet revolution described in this chapter. When this voice did, in fact, permit those at functional levels to influence the decisions that directly affected their work situation, social cohesion increased, and was visible in increased morale and motivation. When this "voice" was mere democratic gesturing about decisions that already had been made, morale and motivation were not increased, and in some instances a decrease in morale was expressed in such things as increased absenteeism and an increase in the production of scrap. Even though such innovation was not, in the first instance, a systematic attempt to decentralize decision-making, it did, in fact, do so in those cases in which the desired results were obtained.

In 1941, I made an interesting mistake, and I am going to use that mistake to show how industry could begin to change its decision-making patterns without realizing what it was doing. During 1941, I was experimenting with the working environment of a group of women who were assembling an electrical gadget for airplanes. I wanted to see whether or not certain changes in the worker's physical environment would increase their output. During this experiment I did a number of things to produce an experiment in the worker's social environment without realizing what I was doing.

What did I change in the physical environment? I changed such things as the color of the walls and the equipment, the level of the noise, the amount of carbon dioxide in the air, and the chairs on which the workers sat. I was gratified to find that each "improvement" in the physical environment increased output. When I had satisfied myself that "improvements" in the physical environment increased output, I put my finding to a further test by systematically introducing adverse changes in the physical environment. I "worsened" the workers' environment by introducing such things as fatigue-producing chairs, and by increasing carbon dioxide to its previous level. To my complete surprise the workers' output continued to rise. I had accidently triggered the "Hawthorne effect." [2] This phenomenon makes it difficult for social scientists to determine whether the results of their experiments are due to their experimental variables, or to enhancements in the social environment.

When I examined my field notes, I was able to discover what had happened. Two significant changes in the worker's social environment had been made. The experimental workers had been incorporated into the decision-making process, and they had ceased to be almost anonymous members of a female work force which numbered, at that time, well over 20,000 persons. At the beginning of the experiment, I had approached the workers, and asked them if they would work with me on a project in which there would be no piece work. They decided to participate. We decided together that a flat rate of time and one-half would be fair to them and to the firm. This rate was selected because the Time Study Department and the "banking system" both used this rate as a "ceiling." The

---

[2] The Hawthorne effect of "halo" is reported in numerous papers published about the so-called Hawthorne studies. One classic account is: F. J. Roethlishenger and W. J. Dickson, *Management and the Worker* (Cambridge, Mass.: Harvard University Press, 1939).

workers made all the decisions about tea and meal breaks and about how the work on the unit was to be organized.

They did not decide what environmental changes were to be made, and they did not know why the changes that they could see were being made. But it was clear that they felt privileged because a number of visible changes were made. Even when they recognized some of these changes as a change for the worse, they felt privileged because the firm was paying special attention to them. Their comments when their fatigue-reducing chairs were replaced by fatigue-producing chairs made this perfectly clear. It was also clear that they felt that through me they had a voice at high levels in the organization; I had arranged for the pay rates that *we* had decided to ask for. The fact that the managing director periodically came into the unit to talk with me supported this assumption.

I have described my own accidental experiment in decentralized decision-making in considerable detail because the revolution in large-scale organization that is mentioned at the beginning of this chapter began in this same accidental manner. Industry was not consciously changing its decision-making patterns. This change began as a by-product of schemes designed to improve morale and motivation. Schemes like this are now being introduced into hospital management. In addition, an innovation in nursing organization has begun to create this same kind of patchy revolution. I will use the innovation in nursing organization to demonstrate the dynamics of changing decision-making patterns in a hospital setting.

This new way of organizing hospital nurses is called the unit-manager system. Numerous modifications of this system are to be found. The system described in this chapter was the first such innovation to persist. Previous attempts by other hospitals had been abandoned. Thus, the unit-manager system described here can be thought of as the parent innovation. This innovation separates the traditional responsibilities of the head nurse into two parts: the management of patient-care and the management of the patient-care unit. The management of the unit is seen as an administrative function. The responsibility for administrative matters is placed under a lay person with administrative skills, and this person is made directly responsible to a superior office in hospital administration. This lay person is called a unit manager, and he or she employs a staff of other lay people to do all the tasks that need to be done in order to make the patient-care unit a place where the nurse can care for patients while physicians are attempting to cure them. The unit manager is responsible for such things as seeing to it that supplies are ordered, drugs are ordered, meals are provided, equipment is available, forms are filled, telephones are answered, and so forth. In short, the unit manager sees to it that the business end of the operation is attended to.

In this system nursing is organized in a new manner. The responsibility for the management of patient-care is placed under *one* nurse who is responsible for the patient-care on her unit twenty-four hours a day for 365 days a year. The nurse in charge of patient-care on a unit is directly responsible to the Director of Nursing Service, and she delegates responsibility to service team leaders. On a sixty-four bed unit, there are three service team leaders. Each service team leader is a clinical specialist responsible for the management of the nursing-care of a patient-population with specialized complaints: neurological complaints, orthopedic complaints, and so forth. Each service team leader is responsible for the nursing-care of her specialized patient-population twenty-four hours a day for 365 days a year. The service team leader has three teams of nursing persons, one for each eight-hour shift. Each of these teams is managed by a nursing team leader who is responsible for the nursing-care given to the patients during the shift when she is on duty. The director of Nursing Service is responsible at all times for the patient-care in the entire hospital, and she does not have the traditional staff of assistants functioning out of her office. She does have a staff assistant responsible to her for in-service education, but this person does not have administrative authority.

The unit-manager system complicates the task of coordinating ward functions by introducing a third factor, an administrative arm. In the traditional situation, conflicts about the ward were fought out between the physicians and the nurses, with the administrator backing whichever contestant it was most expedient for him to back at any particular moment. When the administrator has a staff directly responsible to his office on each patient-care unit, he is forced to alter his tactics because he is no longer entirely free to play the balance of power game.

When this innovation was first introduced, those who designed it realized that it would be cumbersome to permit conflicts that could be resolved on the ward, to work their way up three chains of command, seeking resolution in superior offices. For this reason the unit-manager system was designed to decentralize decision-making to a functional level. In theory at least, the three separate ward functions are coordinated by the cooperative actions of the chief resident, the nurse in charge, and the unit manager.

Within each patient-care unit where decision-making patterns have been effectively decentralized, there is good morale and high motivation. These units look and act like well-integrated and extremely cohesive, small hospitals. They have all the advantages of being small without the disadvantages. They function as if they were small systems, and all the resources of a large institution are available to them. The development of a number of small, independent-minded systems within a large institution that was originally organized in a bureaucratic manner has produced interesting adjustments and fascinating problems. I will describe some of these adjustments and problems in order to show how the decision-making patterns of the institution were altered.

Nursing's decision-making patterns were most radically altered because nursing drastically changed its supervision patterns. It is not easy for a nurse who has been trained to function in a traditional manner to learn how to supervise patient-care when she is not physically present. At first the nurse in charge spent more than a working week in the hospital, and she tended to develop an informal head-nurse system to which she delegated authority. As this nurse became comfortable about being responsible when she was not in the hospital, she began to develop a functional style that enabled her to meet the unique nursing-management problems of her own patient-care units. During this initial phase, her other major problem was developing a productive relationship with the unit manager. The nurse had to learn to have confidence in a lay person's ability to discharge responsibilities that formerly belonged to the head nurse. The traditional head-nurse patterns of thought, action, and decision-making were difficult to change.

As soon as this first phase was over, it became possible for the nurse in charge to help her service-team leaders to function in a flexible manner and to supervise and organize the nursing care of each specialized patient population. This meant that the team leaders were the only nurses with any nursing management responsibilities who functioned in a somewhat traditional manner. As one would expect, these radical changes in nursing organization have tended to breed further decentralization. On some of the patient-care units team leaders and staff nurses have decentralized the responsibility for individual patients. These nurses still work the traditional shift, and while they are on duty they work as a team to care for all the patients on the unit, but the responsibility for planning and supervising the care of individual patients is now divided up among all the registered nurses. Each patient now has his or her nurse, and the nurse holds herself responsible if her patients do not get adequate care.

Although Nursing Service's organizational style was most radically changed when the unit-manager system was introduced some interesting changes were demanded from hospital administration. The most striking change was the assumption of responsibility for institutional slack. Hospital administration's new arm became responsible for bridging the gaps in service that occur at night, during week ends, and on holidays—in the traditional situation the nurse takes up institutional slack. Administration found this new demand relatively easy to adjust to. The most difficult adjustment, interestingly enough, was learning to seek and to accept information about the units from their own lay managers. Hospital administrators are in the habit of relying on nurses for much of the information on which administrative decisions are based. The administrator frequently decides to buy a piece of equipment for one department, and to refuse the request of another department on the basis of information supplied by his director of Nursing Service.

My comments in the preceding paragraphs have particular reference to the in-patient units. In the clinics, in other parts of the teaching hospital and in the colleges, the unit-manager system is used to relieve professional staff of management functions. This fact enabled me to observe what was to all intents and purposes the same innovation in a number of different situations. The interesting thing was that the same innovation produced different results. In some cases the decision-making patterns were decentralized within the unit administered by the unit manager. In some cases no effective decentralization occurred. And in some cases the decision-making patterns outside the unit administered by the unit manager changed.

There have been two cases in which no effective decentralization occurred, and in both cases the same conditions were present. The incumbent in the office immediately superior to that of the unit manager was unable to delegate either responsibility or authority. In both cases decision-making patterns remained centralized, and the fiction that the unit manager was making the decisions that his job description specified was given occasional lip service.

In those cases in which decentralization characterized the unit but did not go further than the unit, the person to whom the unit manager was directly responsible had difficulty delegating sufficient authority to enable the unit manager to discharge his or her responsibilities. Among those units that fell into this category, one small group of units was particularly interesting. This group of units was responsible to a young man who became disturbed because each unit in his empire had developed its own idiosyncratic functional style. He attempted to correct this flaw by insisting on an *appearance* of uniformity. He developed elaborate systems for keeping the same things in the same places on all units. It was interesting to observe the various ways in which other categories of staff on each of these units cooperated to defeat these attempts to impose surface conformity. When the staff on any one unit felt that their own unit manager was in danger of being penalized for their resistance, the nurses and the physicians would begin to manufacture a case against administration. When they had created a sufficient excuse they would enter the hospital administrator's office to stage the traditional tirade against bureaucratic asininity. These paper-dragon battles always included an opportunity to make it quite clear that *their unit manager* was a paragon of all administrative virtues.

Two opposite circumstances seemed to produce an effective decentralized decision-making system that changed the decision-making patterns in superior offices. In some instances, the immediately superior office was a vacuum. In other instances, the superior officer believed in and was extremely adept at delegating authority. When either of these two circumstances was present, and when the unit manager was a competent person, decision-making was decentralized to the units, and the superior office relinquished its traditional right to make decisions about the domestic policy of the units.

The unit-manager system is merely one innovation that is capable of changing the hospital's decision-making patterns. Many of the newer man-management practices that hospitals are borrowing from industry have the potential to create changes similar to the change described in this chapter. In addition, decentralized management of one kind or another is becoming increasingly fashionable in hospital circles. It is now spoken of as decentralized hospital management and has been adopted in thousands of hospitals, both in this country and abroad.[3] Thus, it is safe to say that the hospital, like other large-scale institutions in America, is changing from a bureaucratic form of organization, and it is tending to become corporate in character. In the next chapter, I will show how and why the hospital invites certain kinds of changes precisely because it is changing in this way.

[3] Information supplied by the Surgeon General's office during the Quail Roost Conference on Decentralized Hospital Management, July 1967.

5

The Hospital Invites Change

In the last chapter, I said that hospitals are changing from a bureaucratic form of organization to a corporate form of organization. This change has merely begun, but it is safe to predict that it will continue. The hospital's habit of modeling itself on big business is sufficient guarantee. In this chapter, I intend to examine the hospital's tolerance for innovation, and to suggest various ways in which patient-care might be improved by making strategic use of the hospital's inclination to change in a particular direction.

What happens during change? Change disturbs the status quo; and until a new status quo is established, potential imbalances exist. During these transitional periods, a social system is vulnerable in relationship to the changes it is assimilating. The hospital is changing its decision-making patterns; and until this change has been assimilated, it will be vulnerable in its decision-making processes. The institution's vulnerability will be expressed in three ways. The hospital will tend to accept innovations that decentralize decision-making and other processes. Decision-making boundaries will tend to shift even when new specialities are not emerging. Furthermore, we can expect an increase in boundary fighting.

In previous chapters I have shown how hospitals are beginning to decentralize decision-making to functional levels, and I have described some of the ways in which this particular change demands other changes. I have shown that all categories of hospital specialists establish and defend decision-making territories, and I have suggested some of the ways in which changes in decision-making territories are made. This information permits us not only to identify and characterize the kinds of change that hospital organization can tolerate but also permits us to design changes that will be acceptable to the changing system. Let us suppose that we have decided to design a system of patient-care that is already adapted to the emerging decision-making patterns of the hospital.

What kind of patient-care would we want our new system to produce? We might begin by designing a system that would correct some of the adverse changes that occurred when patient-care was moved from the home into the hospital. When patient-care was administered in the home, the nurse's domain was the sickroom. She inconvenienced the family, and she demanded changes in household behavior in order to maintain the integrity of the sickroom. The sickroom was the patient's therapeutic environment, and the nurse protected her patient's interests by establishing and maintaining an environment that encouraged the patient to respond to treatment and care.

When patient-care was moved from the home to the hospital, the geographical boundaries of the sickroom ceased to be four walls. The patient's therapeutic environment became the wards, the corridors, the elevators, and the treatment and procedure rooms in various parts of the hospital. When patient-care was institutionalized, the patient was placed in "horizontal orbit," and little attention was paid to providing him with a therapeutic environment when he was in any part of the hospital other than on the ward. The contemporary patient spends considerable portions of the hospital day in corridors, elevators, and way-stations.

Another significant change occurred when patient-care was institutionalized. The work of caring for the patient and organizing him into the hospital system was separated into a number of different tasks, and parceled out to a number of different hospital specialists. The result, as far as the patient is concerned, is that he sometimes feels that he is being cared for by a number of differently specialized people who never talk to each other about his problems and his needs. He gets this impression for two reasons. In most hospitals the various hospital specialists responsible for caring for and attempting to cure him do not get together and decide how the resources of the hospital should be used to meet the needs of their patients. This lack of coordination frequently becomes obvious to the patient. That the patient is asked to answer the same questions over and over again leads him to suspect that those who care for him never speak to each other about him and about his problems. The contemporary patient is cared for by a group of task-oriented specialists. This group of skills is called the health team, presumably on the assumption that those who work around the same patients and in the same building automatically become a team. This assumption is not well founded.

A task-oriented approach to patient-care produces a potential for gaps in patient-care. Some years ago, I went into a patient's room during breakfast. The bedfast patient was trying to reach the bedside table which had been left a few inches out of her reach. On top of the table was a wastepaper basket, and on top of the basket was a breakfast tray. I could see a stack of pancakes on which the butter was melting, and I could smell the coffee as I came through the doorway. I was looking at a gap in patient-care. The maid had cleaned the room and forgotten to remove the wastepaper basket and position the bedside table. The waitress had obeyed *her* instructions to place the tray as close to its proper place as possible without interfering with anything in the room, including the patient. The patient told me that the waitress had explained that she had been instructed not to touch the wastepaper basket, move the table, or call a nurse. She had left promising to speak to a friend who worked as an aide on the unit. Gaps in patient-care are not always as visible as the one described above, but a task-oriented system of organizing patient-care can be counted on to exercise its potential for creating gaps.

When patient-care was moved into the hospital the patient lost his traditional defender, the nurse. The sickroom lost its former geographical boundaries, and the nurse continued to think of the therapeutic environment as if it were confined within a single set of four walls. The nurse did not feel responsible for the patient when he was not under her immediate jurisdiction. As a consequence, she did not feel that it was her place to see to it that the patient's therapeutic environment was maintained in all parts of the hospital. No other category of hospital specialist has moved into this vacuum, and the contemporary patient has no one to speak out on his behalf.

Another adverse change in patient-care occurred: the nurse lost the patient. When the nurse and patient-care were institutionalized, the nurse began to work with other nurses and nursing persons to care for the same patient-population and to speak of these patients as the "patient load." Under these circumstances, the nurse ceased to feel as if any particular patient was *her* patient. The loss of a sense of responsibility for individual patients makes it more difficult for the nurse to act as the patient's defender. Nurses frequently want to speak out about conditions that adversely affect their patients, but they have been organized into a position from which it seems impossible to function in this manner. They do not feel, for example, that they have the right to protest against the way in which x-ray departments routinely keep patients waiting for long periods of time in corridors in order to make the maximum use of expensive equipment.

The question is how can we make opportunistic use of the hospital's changing decision-making patterns to introduce a system of patient-care that would correct these adverse changes? How can we give the patient the impression that he is being cared for and cared about by a team of specialists who get together and decide together how to solve his problems? How can the nurse regain her sense of responsibility for individual patients and reassume her traditional role as patient-protector? How can we see to it that the patient's environment is therapeutic while he is in "horizontal orbit"? And how can we remove the potential gaps in patient-care?

Nursing's continuous responsible presence in the hospital and close to the patient places the nurse in a strategic position to correct most of these adverse changes. If nursing were to attempt to develop such a remedial program, an obvious beginning would be to move in three directions. Changes could be made within the nurse's existing decision-making territories. The nurse could occupy territories that have not been claimed by other specialities. In addition, the possibility that some of the existing gaps in patient care are the result of gaps between existing decision-making territories could be considered.

If this approach were to be used, one would look first at the changes that would need to be made in the nurse's functional style in those areas where the nurse's right to make decisions would not be challenged. What could be done on the wards, in the elevators, and in the corridors to establish the image of the nurse as the person who speaks out on the patient's behalf? In these areas, the nurse would be relatively free to take any action that would be to the best interests of her patients. It would be much easier to decide what action was needed if the nurse began by reestablishing her sense of responsibility for individual patients. The simple expedient of making each registered nurse responsible for planning and supervising the care of particular patients even though she continued to work with all the patients, would accomplish this result. Once established as the patient's nurse, the nurse is in a position to become the patient's protector, and to speak out on his behalf.

Common sense suggests that the image of the nurse as a person who speaks out on the patient's behalf should be established first in the no-man's land of elevators and corridors and in the nurse's recognized domain, the ward. Any change in these areas that would seem to decrease patient-stress would be either feebly fought or welcomed by other categories of hospital worker. As far as elevators and corridors are concerned, action by the nurse would relieve a generalized feeling of uneasiness about the conditions that sometimes are encountered in these unclaimed areas. As far as the ward is concerned, gaps in patient-care might command the nurse's immediate attention. It would not be necessary to take drastic action. A policy of common sense would have encouraged the person from dietary to do what she wanted to do, which was to remove the wastepaper basket, and to position the bedside table before she deposited the breakfast tray. Many gaps in patient-care exist merely because unskilled and semi-skilled workers are not permitted to use common sense. The limits within which common sense should be exercised could be clearly defined so that mere common sense would not intrude into areas where clinical judgments must be made. Another possibility would be to partially decentralize centralized service departments. Janitors, housemaids, dietary maids, and couriers could be regrouped, made multifunctional, and placed under the direction of patient-care units. This change tends to increase the morale of these workers.

The patient's sense of being divided into different tasks that are assigned to a number of different people who never talk to each other would decrease if each nurse were to assume responsibility for individual patients. This shift from responsibility for a patient load to responsibility for individual patients invariably increases the nurse's communication with the patient's physician and with others who work with the patient. This increase in communication is obvious to the patient, and he begins to feel that the nurse is coordinating the team of specialists who are working on his behalf. The patient is right: communication makes those who work with the same patient into a team, and the person who communicates directly with *all* members of the team does, in a sense, coordinate it.

When no-man's land had been annexed and after patient-care gaps on the ward had been attended to, a precedent would have been established. The nurse would have created a new image. She would be seen by other categories of hospital workers as the person who defends the patient's therapeutic interests at all times and in all parts of the hospital. When the nurse has reestablished her traditional function as patient-protector, it would be reasonable to assume that stress-producing practices in other departments could be questioned and modified. Such things as stacking patients at the entrances to the rooms occupied by expensive equipment is an excellent example of a thoughtless practice that produces patient-stress.

For instance, x-ray departments do not intend to increase patient-stress by keeping patients waiting in corridors. They are merely organizing their operation in a rational manner. X-ray departments tend to focus their attention on the maximum use of expensive equipment, and the easiest way to make economic use of an x-ray machine is to stockpile patients. X-ray departments routinely schedule on a miniumum time-per-procedure basis, and those who work in these departments sometimes are unaware that waiting to be x-rayed can be, and frequently is, a stress-producing experience. When I talked to radiologists about this matter they were surprised. One department head said: "No one has ever raised this issue."

The nurse is in a unique position to raise such an issue, and to insist that the physical and social environment available to each patient should be as therapeutic as possible. The hospital environment is imposed on the patient, and in some cases he is victimized by it. The hospital's social and physical environment is not an inevitable way of life into which each patient must be crammed or stretched. The hospital is changing, and the environment of the hospital patient can be changed. It *is* possible to modify the hospital environment to meet the therapeutic needs of the patient-population. The patient's hospital environment need not be merely an arbitrarily imposed way of institutionalized life. It can become a consciously contrived way back to life and health. It seems to me that it is a proper function of the nursing profession to see to it that such a change is made.

The nurse, because of nursing's continuous responsible presence on the ward, is in a superior position to see to it that the patient's environment is therapeutic at all times, in all parts of the hospital. However, the nurse cannot make this change single-handed. All hospital specialists have a responsibility to make the patient's environment as therapeutic as possible. The nurse may insist that the therapeutic interests of the patient come first, but unless all categories of hospital specialists are prepared to act on this assumption, the nurse's insistence will not produce the changes that are needed. The hospital cannot cease to be a place in which the patient's needs are met at the convenience of machines and specialized people, until all those who work in hospitals recognize their tendency to turn their means into ends. When means are turned into ends, the hospital patient becomes the "low man on the totem pole." When this happens, the hospital begins to act as if it could function more effectively if it could diagnose, treat, and care for things rather than for people. Having looked at the hospital in some detail, we will next look at the person who makes hospitals necessary: the patient.

Part   Two

HOSPITAL ROLES
AND RELATIONSHIPS

6

The Hospital Patient

After I had completed my study of the hospital as a social system, I
returned to the patient-care units to look at the various categories of
persons in it. I looked first at the patient: partly because hospitals are
organized to benefit patients; and partly because I already was curious
about why those who work in hospitals label patients "good" and "bad."
The first thing I found was that staff members, aides, nurses, physicians,
and other hospital specialists, rarely volunteered it as their opinion that
so-and-so was a "good" patient, but when a patient had earned the opposite
label, they referred to him as a "bad" patient when they talked with each
other about him. This meant that, unless I was prepared to make the staff
self-conscious about the way in which they categorized patients as "good"
and "bad," I would be well advised to begin my examination of how
those who work in hospitals expect their patients to behave by collecting
information about the behavior of "bad" patients.

At the end of seven months, I had detailed information about 169
patients. In this collection twenty-three were "good" patients, sixty-nine
were "good" patients who had turned "bad," and seventy-seven were

"bad" patients. The twenty-three "good" patients were identified by various staff members during attempts to make me understand why they, the staff, thought of and spoke about particular patients as "bad" patients. The following incident suggests how "good" patients got into my "bad" patient collection:

> Mrs. B earned the "bad" patient label because she "sneaked off the unit to talk with her three-year-old." I had talked with Mrs. B before the nurse told me what Mrs. B had done to earn the "bad" patient label. Mrs. B said: "I did not know that I would not be able to go into the waiting room, and I had told Linda that she could visit me in the hospital while I was away having the baby. I thought it best to risk angering the staff than to disappoint my daughter." After I explained to the nurse why Mrs. B had done what she did, the nurse said: "Mrs. C (another new mother) wanted to see her children as much if not more so. Mrs. C is a 'good' patient and Mrs. B a 'bad' one."

The "good" patients who turned into "bad" patients were not identified as such until they had developed what those who work in hospitals refer to as "hospitalitis," an apparent desire to remain in the hospital after the physician has informed the patient that he is well enough to go home. A staff nurse described a typical case of "hospitalitis" in the following manner:

> Yesterday, Mr. T was ready to go home, and he seemed pleased when the physician told him that he was to be discharged this morning. He gave the night and evening girls a dreadful time. He couldn't sleep, he complained of pain, and he insisted that they call his doctor. Of course, they knew what the matter was: Mr. T likes it here and wants to stay. This morning Mr. T's physician said: "We'd better keep him here for two or three days and run some more tests." Mr. T was a "good" patient, now we're going to have difficulty getting him out of the hospital.

The patients who became "bad" patients earlier in the hospital stay, rather than at the news that it was to be terminated, were described as: asking too many questions; refusing to do what they were told to do; insisting on "carrying on" from the hospital bed as if they were either at home or in their offices, and making what the staff considered excessive demands. The following were among the examples of patients who behaved in these ways:

> The colostomy in 543 refuses to take his medication until he is told what it is, and why he has to take it.

> Mrs. K asks too many questions. She's on vital signs every two hours, and even though we have told her over and over again that we can't tell her, she keeps asking what her temperature is. And every time she has a bowel movement, she wants to know whether it is satisfactory or not. She's been in two weeks and she ought to know by this time that we cannot answer questions of this kind.

Mr. F's secretary comes in twice a day and sits there, bold as brass, taking dictation. A hospital room is not an office.

His light is always on and when you go in to find out what he wants, it's something he could do without. He acts as if we didn't have other patients to look after, and most of them are sicker than he is.

I used the information suggested thus far in this chapter to characterize the role that those who work in hospitals seem to expect their patients to play.

The role is temporary. There is no such thing as a permanent hospital patient. Sooner or later, the patient is dischargd, either back into society or into another institution, or he dies. In most cases the temporariness of the role is invoked abruptly. It is usual practice not to forewarn the patient. The physician is not absolutely sure when his patient will be ready for discharge, and he prefers not to raise false hopes. The patients who developed "hospitalitis" had been sufficiently submissive and undemanding to be thought of, in retrospect, as "good" patients until they fell from grace by producing a new crop of symptoms as soon as the physician told them that they were about to be discharged from the hospital. I began to wonder whether the incidence of "hospitalitis" could be reduced if patients were prepared for discharge well in advance. Later in this chapter I will describe an attempt to experiment with this notion.

All other reasons for labeling patients "bad" suggested two characteristics of the hospital patient's role. He is expected to submit himself to the rules and regulations of the institution and to the decisions of its specialists; and he is expected to relinquish his real-life responsibilities even when he is capable of discharging them from the hospital bed. If he asks questions, refuses to do what he is asked to do unless he is told why, demands more attention than the staff thinks he needs, and if he tries to discharge his responsibilities to his family and his job, he is likely to be considered a "bad" patient. I thought of the patients who earned a bad reputation in these four ways as too independent-minded for the system to tolerate, and I began to realize that the staff's expectation of patient behavior was contradictory in nature. On the one hand, the patient is expected to instantly become totally dependent, and to abandon all responsibilities other than those directly connected with his illness. On the other hand, he is expected to become independent rapidly enough to leave the hospital at short notice. As soon as I became aware of the possible contradictions in the hospital patient's role, I decided to interview staff and patients.

The staff was asked to describe the ideal patient, a question that produced descriptions of patients who were submissive, undemanding, and when the time came to do so, delighted to leave the hospital. In some cases these descriptions included an additional ingredient: that the patient appreciate what has been done for him. Next they were asked to describe their most rewarding experiences with individual patients. The third question was about frustrating experiences with patients. The staff's rewarding experiences with patients described situations in which the patient did better than the staff had expected. The patient recovered against odds, the patient responded rapidly to treatment, and so forth. The frustrating experiences, on the other hand, tended to be descriptions of situations in which the patient did not respond to treatment and care as vigorously as the staff had anticipated. The physicians interviewed had an additional category of frustrating experiences: the patient whom they could not satisfactorily diagnose. They also had an additional rewarding category: the diagnosis against odds.

As a direct consequence of these interviews, I began to speculate with the staff about the differences between patients who responded to treatment in a rewarding manner and patiens who did not. The staff came to the conclusion that the independent mindedness, which under certain circumstances earned the "bad" patient label, was a valuable characteristic when it was channeled in the right direction. Refusal to submit might make a patient difficult to handle, but it could make a vital difference to his ability to recover. The staff also decided that the patients who seemed to welcome the opportunity to be dependent on others tended to recover slowly. These discussions raised an interesting question: Is it therapeutically sound to insist that all patients become as submissive and dependent as the hospital's traditional expectations demand?

Interviews with patients were conducted in a leisurely manner, and each informant was given an opportunity to volunteer to answer this four-part question: What is *your* idea of a "good" doctor, a "good" nurse, a "good" patient, and a "good" hospital? Three hundred and sixty-five patients and their visitors were questioned in this indirect manner, in some cases by me, in other cases by a nurse. The information from these conversations was interesting. The most striking fact was that the patients had two different sets of responses. Almost half of them seemed to want an omniscient doctor and a submissive patient-role. The other half seemed to want a doctor with skill and knowledge and a cooperative patient-role.

The patients who wanted the traditional role seemed uneasy when the "good" hospital was under consideration. When they were asked to make suggestions about improving the hospital, they either shied away from the topic or offered platitudes about how nice everything and everyone was. The patients who seemed to want a cooperative role had clearcut ideas about the "good" hospital, and they made sensible suggestions about how the hospital could be improved.

Interestingly enough, we did not get a clear picture of the "good" nurse from more than a handful of our informants. Attempts to secure a volunteered definition of the "good" nurse produced either platitudes about the hospital's wonderful nurses, or complaints about specific nursing practices. The patients resisted describing the "good" nurse even when the interviewer was not a nurse. At a later date, I attempted to discover why these 365 patients seemed to avoid describing the "good" nurse, and I came to an interesting conclusion.

Nursing's continuous responsibility for the patient-care unit gives the nurse situational authority over the life-style of the patient. During the hospital stay, the patient feels that it is unwise to make candid comments about those who seem to him to have unlimited opportunities to deny his requests and ignore his needs. As soon as the patient has been discharged from the hospital, he is willing to describe the "good" nurse, and to give concrete examples of what he thinks of as "bad" nursing. In retrospect, the hospital patient values competent physical care, being made to feel that he is not imposing on the nurse, and the sense of being understood and valued as a person.

Interviews with hospital patients suggested that patients would like two roles: a submissive role and a cooperative role. Those at lower socioeconomic levels, and those in critical condition seem to want an omniscient doctor and a submissive patient-role. Those at higher socioeconomic levels, and those who are not in critical condition seem to want a cooperative patient-role. Just over 5 percent of the patients interviewed shifted their preferences during the course of the hospital stay. These shifts were not in the same direction, but they were inevitably accompanied by either a marked change in the patient's condition or a marked change in the patient's perception of his condition. This kind of change dramatically alters the patient's stress and anxiety levels. When stress and anxiety increased rapidly, the patient who had previously desired a cooperative role would embrace the submissive role. When stress and anxiety decreased rapidly, a submissive patient tended to seek the cooperative role.

Two sets of responses about the role of hospital patient and the tendency to shift from one role to another when the patient's stress and anxiety level changes rapidly suggest that the traditional role has become obsolete, and should be replaced by a role in which absolute submissiveness is replaced by an independent-dependent continuum. If this were done, the absolute insistence that the hospital patient abandon his usual responsibilities could be replaced by a responsibility continuum. Those who are capable of discharging some of their usual responsibilities from the hospital bed could be permitted to do so.

During our study of the patient-role, we consistently used one question that we thought of as an ice-breaker. The question was: What do you miss most? Those who seemed to want an omniscient doctor and a submissive patient-role invariably said that they most missed some material comfort, tobacco, particular foods, their own pillow, and so forth. Those who seemed to want a cooperative patient-role, on the other hand, invariably said that they most missed people and activities. Those who reversed themselves on the patient-role, simultaneously changed what they said they missed. The fact that when a patient seemed to want a dependent role, he missed creature comforts, and that when he wanted a cooperative role, he missed his associates and activities suggested a simple way in which the nurse and other hospital specialists could determine whether the patient needed to be dependent or independent at any particular moment.

The possibility of determining the role-needs of each patient in a relatively simple manner raised a new question. Would it be feasible to permit hospital patients to play two different roles, and if so, could these two different roles be contained in the same room or ward? I had no difficulty finding nurses interested in exploring this possibility. Five nurses began to experiment with this possibility. They found that they were able to permit their patients to choose either one of these two roles. They also found that it was possible for them to do so even when the patients playing the two different roles occupied adjacent beds in the same room.

These five nurses carried my findings even further. They became interested in the possibility of decreasing the hospitalitis rate by preparing the naturally submissive patient for discharge well in advance. They explained that in some cases, a patient has little notice of discharge. They felt that if some days before discharge, they began to prepare all those patients who most missed material comforts, they could decrease the hospitalitis rate. They discussed this plan with the physicians, and both the physicians and the nurses worked together to implement the plan. During the three months that I watched this particular experiment, there was only one case of hospitalitis among the patients that these five nurses cared for.

My examination of the hospital patient's role suggested that two of its characteristics can, and possibly should, be expanded into continuums, and that hospitalitis tends to decrease when the patient who is unsure of his ability to function after he has left the hospital is prepared for discharge well in advance. During the course of this particular study, I also collected information about the social desirability of the hospital patient's role, and I did so for two reasons: the sick role is socially undesirable in that it deprives society of the services of the sick person, and burdens it with his care; and because the role of hospital patient originally was a role for a critically ill person unable to pay for the care he needed. I found an interesting hierarchy of social desirabilities.

Those with communicable diseases are stigmatized because these diseases are dangerous to others and in this sense are antisocial. They also make more work for those who must care for them.[1] If the communicable disease is considered an inevitable part of growth and development, one of the so-called childhood diseases, and if the victim is an appropriate age, the social stigma of having it tends to be balanced out. Venereal diseases carry an added stigma because they suggest that the patient is no better than he should be. Resourcelessness and irresponsible behavior add stigma to any disease, and a patient who has been brought to the hospital from a prison is stigmatized even when he has a socially desirable diagnosis. In our society, it is considered socially desirable to give birth to babies in hospitals, and to do so on the way to the hospital inconveniences the hospital, and makes the woman who has done so seem less desirable than she otherwise would have been. If unorthodox delivery occurs in the Admission Office, the patient's social reputation is enhanced because those who work with her after she reaches the hospital bed tend to feel that the Admission Office processes their patients in an unnecessarily leisurely manner. Delivery Room nurses frequently are overheard saying such things as "It would serve them right if someone delivered at the desk" (in the Admission Office).

There are other ways in which the patient-role can become socially desirable. Complaints to which those with valued traits are thought to be particularly prone become prestigeful complaints—ulcers, for example. Conditions that are courted during valued activities add luster to the patient-role: the injuries characteristically courted by football players fall into this category. Diagnostic categories that provide opportunities for conspicuous consumption make the patient role socially desirable: elaborate check-ups and elective surgery produce excellent examples. As one would have expected, moving a cross section of society into the role of hospital patient has changed the social undesirability of that role into a hierarchy of relative desirabilities which reflect the value system of our society. It is socially undesirable to be sick, but in some cases more so than in others.

I summarized my study of the hospital patient by making the following comments in my field diary:

> Hospital patients fall into two categories: those who would welcome the opportunity to play a cooperative role, and those who are prepared to submit themselves to the role that the hospital seems to expect them to play.
>
> Those patients who would prefer a cooperative role are willing to submit their diseases to the jurisdiction of physicians, and they are willing to accommodate themselves to what they consider to be the reasonable

---

[1] Patients with communicable diseases are isolated, and time-consuming precautions are taken to see to it that their germs are not carried to other patients.

demands of the hospital and its specialists. They resent being treated as if they were incompetent, and they do not hesitate to outwit the system when an opportunity arises. When they are capable of doing so, they would like to cooperate with those who are caring for them. They want to understand what is happening to them, and they are inclined to believe that they would respond more rapidly to treatment if they were permitted to become active participants.

Those who seek and are prepared to submit to the submissive patient-role seem to fall into four categories. Patients who temporarily are incapable of managing for themselves. Persons who have been culturally conditioned to believe that submissiveness is an inevitable part of hospitalization: those from lower socioeconomic levels tend to fall into this category. Patients who consider themselves in jeopardy: some minority groups produce patients who feel that they will be injured unless they behave in a conciliatory manner. And those who value a dependent role, and welcome any invitation to become dependent on others.

My study of the hospital patient did not seem complete because I had not found a satisfactory answer to the question: What is a good nurse? Therefore, I decided to talk with discharged patients before I examined the various ways in which the hospital orients the sick person to his role as hospital patient. This digression made me aware of a process that I had not previously thought to examine. As you will see, it was worth discovering and studying because it helped me to understand the hospital patient.

When I followed patients into the community to seek an answer to the question: What is a good nurse?—I became aware of a phenomenon that I had observed for a number of years without realizing what I had been looking at. I had taken it for granted that adults in the society, including myself, consulted a physician when they considered themselves sick enough to do so, and I had not paid particular attention to the interchanges that precede decisions of this sort. My conversations with discharged patients and their families in most cases became descriptions of what had happened to the patient and his family, and these descriptions invariably contained an account of the way in which close friends and family members had participated in making the initial decision to seek out the physician. It soon became obvious that what I was listening to were descriptions of a process that began with a decision to seek cure, and ended when the sick person was readmitted to his usual roles as a well person. I then began to think of this process as cure-seeking behavior. I will present the conclusions I reached after I had analyzed the first hundred descriptions.

The decision to seek help from the physician is preceded by a social drama that turns a physical crisis into a social crisis by making those close to the sick person partners in the decision to consult the physician. Although the physical crisis that precipitates this decision varies from individual to individual and from situation to situation, the drama that precedes the decision to consult a physician serves the same purpose, and is played out in a similar manner whenever a decision to seek medical help is made. A sick person does not consult a physician lightly even when the sickness is slight.

Decisions to consult a physician may seem to have been made either by the sick person or by those close to the sick person, but when we examine the behavior that characteristically precedes these decisions, it becomes clear that both the sick person and those close to him are parties to the decision to seek medical help. Considerable pressure may be exerted by neighbors and acquaintances; but, unless the sickness is recognized as a threat to society, legal pressure is not brought to bear and the right to decide to seek cure is firmly located *around* the sick person. The physician scrupulously maintains the appearance of not interfering in this particular decision.

When a sickness seems serious enough to warrant consulting a physician, it has become a physical crisis, and the cure-seeking behavior that characteristically precedes the decision to turn the sickness over to the physician recognizes the physical crisis in the sick person as a social crisis in the segment of society to which the sick person belongs. When it seems appropriate to seek cure, those closest to the sick person help him to place his sickness under the jurisdiction of the physician. Even when the sick person is capable of acting without assistance, he tends to invite those closest to him to become partners in his decision to seek medical help.

Most of us need to be encouraged to consult a physician even when our symptoms are relatively severe. This becomes clear when we compare the way in which we make decisions to consult the physician with the way in which we make other equally weighty decisions. A university professor first drew my attention to this phenomenon when he told me that he made academic decisions and the decision to consult a physician in a somewhat different manner. He said that he made decisions about the grades he would give and the papers he would present without consulting others, and that he took full responsibility for these decisions; but that if he woke up with a sore throat and felt that he ought to consult his physician about it, he behaved as if he were incapable of making the decision to do so.

> When I wake with a sore throat, I decide either to ignore it, cure it myself, or that it might be wise to consult my physician. My response is dictated by the severity of the symptom, and by the way in which I have been culturally conditioned to respond to a sore throat. If I decide to cure it myself, I take a couple of aspirin tablets, and I do not mention that I have a sore throat unless I wish to draw attention to the splendid way I carry on even when I'm not a well man. If I have decided that it would be wise to consult a physician, I behave quite differently. I take

aspirin, and I make sure that my wife and the children know about it. They suggest that I call the doctor. I resist their suggestion by playing down the severity of my symptoms, but I begin to act as if my throat is much sorer than I am willing to admit. I take a bite of toast, swallow it with obvious difficulty, put the rest of the piece down, and I begin to toy with my breakfast. My family responds to this maneuver by insisting that I am much sicker than I will admit. At first I fight this suggestion vigorously, then I begin to give ground; and when I eventually leave the house, I do so promising that for their sakes I will stop by, and let my physician take a look at my throat.

This ritualized cure-seeking behavior drew attention to what the professor had decided might be a physical crisis, and he turned it into a social crisis, by making those close to him partners in his decision to seek medical help. It also irritated his wife who said: "He makes a dreadful fuss; I wish he would behave sensibly like the rest of us. My daughters and I go to the doctor whenever it seems wise to do so, and nobody has to nag us into it." The professor's wife did not seem to understand that men in our society are expected to resist admitting that they are sick enough to seek help.

The professor recognized a physical crisis, and he drew this crisis to the attention of his family. He involved his family in the decision to seek medical help by resisting their suggestion that he consult a physician. Stylized resistance and insistance continued until the professor's physical crisis had been established as a social crisis in the professor's household, and until the professor had staged a culturally appropriate male response to sickness. It is interesting to observe the relationship between visible symptoms and this traditional struggle. For example, when a sore throat is accompanied by swollen glands and a fever that can be made visible on the thermometer, the ritualized resistance to the suggestion that cure should be sought decreases dramatically.

When a sickness seems severe enough to warrant seeking medical help, ritualized cure-seeking behavior is used to turn the physical crisis into a social crisis. The circumstances that make it seem appropriate to seek medical help vary according to age, sex, and socioeconomic status as well as according to the severity of the symptoms. Just as the appropriate reasons for seeking cure vary from situation to situation, acceptable cure-seeking behavior varies from one situation to another. In order to show some of these variations, we will use the professor's sore throat as our presenting symptom, but we will change the person who has it.

If the sort throat had belonged to a woman not responsible for the care of young children rather than to a man, the initial resistance to the suggestion that a physician be consulted would not have needed to be vigorous. In our society, the woman is thought to be the weaker sex. The devoted mother, on the other hand, is expected to refuse to be sick if it is at all possible to do so.

If the person with the sore throat were extremely poor, it would not seem appropriate to consult a physician. At this socioeconomic level the sick person would need to be in a critical condition in order to make it seem appropriate to seek medical help. If the sick person was either extremely rich or prominent, a mere visit to the physician's office might not seem a sufficiently elaborate gesture. If the sick person was either very young or very old, a relatively minor complaint would be taken more seriously at any level in the socioeconomic hierarchy. These variations are extremely interesting and, because they are expressions of different lifestyles, they must be taken into consideration by those who care for and attempt to cure the sick.

The limits within which it seems appropriate to seek medical help vary from situation to situation, and the sick person who violates these limits is condemned by neighbors and by associates. If he habitually consults the physician when his condition does not seem to warrant it, he earns the reputation of being a hypochondriac. If he refuses to consult a physician when his age, sex, socioeconomic status, and symptoms make it seem imperative that he do so, he and those closest to him are severely criticized. Under the latter circumstances, those who are not intimately associated with the sick person may take action, particularly when the sick person is a child.

Cure-seeking behavior varies from situation to situation and from subculture to subculture in our society, but it has two common characteristics. There are always limits within which it is socially appropriate to seek cure, and the decision to seek this help is sanctioned by those closest to the sick person. The following description of cure-seeking behavior is an excellent example.

A student described the ritualized cure-seeking behavior in an American university dormitory in the following manner:

> The sick person draws the attention of her roommate or closest friend to her condition. As soon as the sick person suggests that the sickness might be severe enough to warrant a stay in the Infirmary, the sick person places her fate in the hands of this closest person who immediately assembles a council of influential dormitory residents. If a nursing student is available, she is summoned to become the "expert" consultant. The nursing student is given this position even when she has not finished her first nursing course, and even when she does not normally function as an influential person in the dormitory society.

> The council surrounds the sick person's bed, and they discuss her case. The sick person is not expected to speak unless she is asked a direct question. The council is held around the bed whether or not the sick

person remains in the bed. Under certain circumstances she may have to leave it. The sick person does not take part in the final phase of this particular decision-making process. Unless the sick person's condition worsens dramatically, the pros and cons are argued at considerable length. When a decision is reached, an affirmative decision is customary, it is implemented by the bed-side council who inform the authorities, pack the patient's suitcase, and deliver her to the Infirmary.

The physician is approached with considerable ceremony, and he, in turn, approaches the problem that the patient presents with appropriate ritual. The decision-making rights of the physician are clear cut. He is supposed to identify the sickness, and having made this decision, to determine a course of treatment. Once the sickness has been turned over to the physician, it is under his jurisdiction until this responsibility is formally terminated. In most cases, the physician decides that it is no longer necessary for him to remain responsible for the patient's sickness. At this point, he discharges the patient. In rare instances, the patient and those close to him terminate their relationship with the physician. When this happens, we say that the patient acted against medical advice. As long as the sickness remains in the physician's hands, however, he has absolute authority over what is to be done to and for the disease.

Cure-seeking behavior serves two purposes: It makes those close to the sick persons parties to the decision to seek medical help, and it prepares the sick person and those close to him for the temporary adjustments that will be required when the physician's plan for treatment is implemented. As soon as the physician decides what is to be done about the disease, the life-style of the patient and of the social systems to which he belongs are rearranged to accommodate the patient's treatment needs. Discharge places the patient back in social circulation, and relieves those close to him of the obligation to cater to him and to his treatment needs.

The return to normal is not abrupt. Even when the sickness has been slight, the transition is marked by ritualized behavior that terminates the social crisis, and celebrates the end of the physical crisis. The person who was sick and is now well is treated like a returned traveler. He is welcomed, he is invited to describe his adventures, and he is regaled with accounts of the changes that occurred during his absence from his accustomed roles. If the sickness was severe, and if the sick person was removed from his usual surroundings during the course of the sickness, the celebration of the traveler's return tends to be elaborated and prolonged. Sicknesses for which cure is sought provide opportunities for individual dramas in a society in which opportunities like this are few and far between.

As we have seen, the decision to seek cure is merely one phase in a complex social process. Let us think about what happens to the sick person, and to those close to him during each phase of this process. In the first instance, the physical crisis presents itself, in some cases abruptly and with considerable drama, and in other cases, it builds up slowly and unobtrusively. In either case, the sick person's stress and anxiety level rises. When the sick person begins to incorporate those close to him in the decision to seek cure, he mobilizes social support. That those close to him care enough about him to insist that he seek help increases his ability to tolerate stress and anxiety.

When the sickness is turned over to the physician, it is unidentified. Placing the sickness in expert jurisdiction decreases stress and anxiety; but, until the disease is identified, considerable anxiety accumulates. When the problem has been identified, the threat to the sick person becomes concrete. The stress and anxiety level may drop dramatically, or it may rise, depending on the sick person's perception of the threatening nature of his diagnostic predicament. The course of treatment decided upon by the physician also has the potential to change the stress and anxiety level in either direction, and in an equally dramatic manner. Surgery is an excellent example of a treatment that tends to create a rapid rise in stress and anxiety although, in some cases, the decision to use the knife decreases anxiety.

The discharge back into normal social circulation is followed by a readmission ceremony that increases the returning member's sense of belonging, and during this ceremony he has a formal opportunity to add his unique adventure to his identity as a group member. In those cases in which the former patient may be anxious because he has separated himself from the expert assistance that he may need, the ceremony that readmits him to society, helps him to support this increase in anxiety. At the least, the readmission ceremony helps the returned member to reorganize himself, and to reassume his usual responsibilities.

During the entire course of a sickness that becomes serious enough to warrant seeking help from a physician, the sick person's stress and anxiety level is in a continuous state of flux. If the sick person is separated by being in the hospital, an additional set of stresses is invoked. In the next two chapters, we will consider what happens when the sick person becomes a hospital patient. In Chapter 9 we will consider various ways in which those who work in hospitals might increase the patient's ability to tolerate the increases in stress and anxiety that are inevitably associated with hospitalization.

7

The Hospital Patient's
Social Dilemma[1]

When a sick person enters the hospital, he must be turned into a patient. As a patient, he must be prepared for "horizontal orbit." This process is not as simple as it seems. The hospital takes custody of the patient's person, arranges to charge the patient for services rendered, organizes the patient's occupancy of space and use of things, sees to it that the patient is cared for and fed, implements the course of treatment determined by the patient's physician, and schedules the patient's journeys to and from the machines that will be used to diagnose and treat him. In order to prepare itself to discharge these complex responsibilities, the hospital has developed a procedure called the admission procedure. In this chapter we will examine the admission procedure, and we will consider its effect on the patient as a person.

[1] The material in the first half of this chapter which appeared in *Nursing Forum* has been rewritten. C. D. Taylor, "Sociological Sheep Shearing," *Nursing Forum* 1, no. 2 (Spring 1962): 79–89. The second half of the chapter appeared in the *American Journal of Nursing;* minor changes have been made. C. D. Taylor, "The Hospital Patient's Social Dilema," *American Journal of Nursing* 65 (October 1965): 96–99.

Except in an emergency and unless he has contrary information about hospital admission, the sick person approaches the hospital secure in the knowledge that the hospital has prepared itself to accept him as a patient. The decision to enter the hospital has been made, the physician has been assured that a bed is available, the sick person and those close to him have begun to act as if the sick person already has become a hospital patient. Under these circumstances, the new patient's first encounter with the hospital is disquieting.

In most cases there is an initial delay. The new patient is asked to wait his turn, and during this wait the patient and those who accompanied him to the hospital either sit in silence or attempt to make conversation. The initial delay creates the same social awkwardness that occurs when leave-takings are prolonged by unexpected delays in departure time. Leave-taking ceremonies tend to deteriorate when the boat or the train does not depart on time. The summons to the admission interview rescues the new patient from this limbo.

The admission interview can be, and frequently is, disturbing. The hospital is prepared to admit the patient, but in order to code the patient into the system, the hospital needs additional information about the patient and his affairs. The hospital charges for its services on a sliding scale; and in order to be fair to itself and the patient, it needs information about the patient's financial status and insurance coverage. The hospital is preparing itself to take custody of the patient's body and personal effects. Things of value, money, jewelry, and so forth, must be put in a safe place. In addition, the hospital must prepare for the worst: If the patient should become incompetent, the hospital must know to whom it should turn. Or if the patient should die, the hospital must know who will pay the hospital bill and to whom the body and its valuables should be surrendered. During the admission interview, collecting this information takes precedence over the patient's need to be assured that the hospital is ready, willing, and able to care for him. At this point the new patient feels like a traveler with a valid passport and the correct visas who is entering a foreign country during the search for a criminal who is known to be attempting illegal entry with forged papers. The patient is relieved when the admission interview is over, and he is dispatched to the hospital floor.

In most hospitals, the patient is escorted to the floor either by a low-level hospital worker or by a volunteer. In either case, those on escort duty have been cautioned not to give the patient information. The new patient's need for information, and the escort's unwillingness to provide information produce conversations at cross purposes. The patient wants to know where he is going, and when he can expect to eat. His escort may reply with comments about the weather and questions about the patient's gardening practices. If the patient is unsophisticated about hospitals, he may have been removed from the admission interview without knowing whether or not those who came with him have been told that the hospital has decided to keep him. The problem that this particular doubt creates is described in a later section.

Admission to the hospital bed proceeds at a relatively rapid rate. The various systems that supply services to the floor are alerted that room and bed number X now contain patient number Y. In due course food, drugs, and treatments will be provided, and orbits to distant machines will be arranged according to this information. The sick person and his effects are placed in the designated spaces. These spaces and the patient are labeled with the patient's new number, and the patient is considered to have been satisfactorily "filed pending flight orders." Care begins at once with routine tests and taking of vital signs, and with routine cleaning, feeding, and toileting. Treatment cannot begin until the physician writes his orders.

As far as the hospital is concerned, the admission process has been completed, and the hospital is prepared for any contingency. The hospital is now ready to orbit the new patient in accordance with the physician's specifications. Hospital services have been mobilized, the hospital floor has the patient on file, and is caring for him. The system contains sufficient information to permit the hospital to discharge its obligations to the patient, to the patient's family, and to the physician.

As far as the patient and his family are concerned the admission process has had somewhat different consequences. It has separated the patient from his family and from society. It has reduced the patient as a person and it has prepared him for his new role as hospital patient.

THE ADMISSION PROCESS	HOW THIS PROCESS OPERATES TO REDUCE A PERSON TO A PATIENT
A clerk obtains the information needed for processing and classification.	This is the confessional phase: The sick person is under compulsion to divulge private information about himself and his affairs. This intimate information is frequently collected in a semi-public place.
A clerk removes valuables for safekeeping.	The sick person must relinquish all outward signs of position and prestige. He is issued a piece of paper in exchange.
An aide or a volunteer escorts the patient to the "floor."	The aide or volunteer takes the sick person's suitcase; a woman often carries a man's bag. The sick person is wheeled through a maze of corridors to the ward, whether or not he

THE ADMISSION PROCESS	HOW THIS PROCESS OPERATES TO REDUCE A PERSON TO A PATIENT
	walked in. If the sick person has protested at any point up to now, he has begun to learn that the hospital is in complete control and dictates terms.
The floor "manager," nurse or lay administrator, receives the papers and the patient.	On the floor, uniforms and other insignia create an atmosphere of regimented strangeness. The papers about the patient are transferred, and in some cases partially read, before the new patient is spoken to or acknowledged. The implication being that the papers and the messages they convey are more important than the patient.
A nurse or aide takes the patient to his room.	The sick person is now a patient. He has a room and possibly a bed number. His room is his filing space and he may be known more by his room number and his disease than by his name. He may become "the diabetic in 405."
The nurse or aide helps the patient to prepare for bed.	This tends to reduce the patient to the lowest common denominator of the system. All patients are helped to undress whether or not they dressed themselves to come to the hospital. The patient is given a gown which is his hospital uniform. The gown tends to alienate him from himself because he does not feel "right" in it. He would never select such a garment for himself. The cut of the hospital gown—short, wide, and split up the back—forces the patient to stay in bed to cover his nakedness. The patient's uniform does not encourage ambulation. Fantasies about bedpans and bedbaths may further alienate the patient from his usual view of himself.
The nurse or aide checks the patient for medication and removes any that he may have in his possession.	The patient has obviously been administering his own medication. He is no longer considered responsible enough to do so.
The nurse takes vital signs.	The patient is classified as to temperature, pulse, respiration, and blood pressure.

THE ADMISSION PROCESS	HOW THIS PROCESS OPERATES TO REDUCE A PERSON TO A PATIENT
The nurse or aide attaches labels to the spaces occupied by the patient and his effects. Labels are attached to patients and the things they use—urinals and so forth.	The order in which the labeling is usually done suggests that the patient is an inanimate object that must be accounted for. The labeling process finally convinces the patient that he is no longer a responsible person. He has become an object for which the hospital is now responsible. Attaching a label to the patient also suggests that he may, at some future date, be unable to reveal his identity to others.
The nurse leaves the patient to attend to the clinical chart.	As soon as admission to the bed has been attended to, the nurse records the outcome on the chart: time and manner of admittance, TRP, BP, and so on. Instead of getting acquainted with her new patient the nurse leaves him alone in a strange environment. In most cases she does not orient him to the life-style of the new world into which he has been plunged.
The nurse and other hospital specialists return.	From now on the door remains open and the patient no longer controls access to and from his bedroom. Visitors, within the limits imposed by specified time, age, and number, enter at will. Hospital specialists enter and leave at their own discretion to carry out orders, and to do things for and to the patient.

The admission process makes it quite clear to the patient that the hospital has accepted him on its own terms, that it will treat him as an incompetent person and that it expects the patient to submit himself to the rules and regulations of the institution and to the decisions of hospital specialists.

The hospital admission procedure is an excellent example of the mass adjustment techniques that have been developed by industrial societies. Industrial societies practice mass production, and in order to do so they need to develop mass demands and to create massive organizations. Neither of these ends can be achieved unless mass-adjustment techniques are used. The mass-production system serves and is served by people. These people must be adjusted and readjusted as rapidly as possible. As consumers, their tastes must be homogenized, and as producers they must become interchangeable units. To this end, mass-adjustment techniques, variously called advertising, training, orientation, internship, and so forth, have been developed. Although these techniques are called by different names, they have a common purpose. The purpose of mass adjustment is to create interchangeable human units with similar tastes, aspirations, and needs. This purpose is accomplished by replacing an old frame of reference with a new frame of reference; one that has been designed to provide a meaningful context for the desired new attitudes and new behavior.

This method of adapting and redesigning people is similar to the shearing done by sheep farmers, but it differs from sheep shearing in one significant way. The sheep farmer values both the wool and the shorn animal, whereas the "people stripper" values the shape of the person after stripping, and discards everything else. If the person is being stripped into a temporary role, the hospital patient is an excellent example, the old frame of reference is filed away for future use. If the person is being prepared for a permanent role, nurse or physician, conflicting segments of the old frame of reference must be destroyed. The mass-adjustment process could be called sociological sheep shearing, and the various ways in which the hospital's admission procedure operates to reduce a person to a patient is an excellent example of sociological sheep shearing.

The admission procedures used by most contemporary hospitals organize the patient into the system, and orient the sick person to the traditional patient role. As we discovered in an earlier chapter, the traditional patient role is obsolete, and the hospital for which this role was designed has disappeared. Today's patient-population is a cross section of society, and it is no longer productive to treat all patients as if they were socially undesirable. As we shall see, it is both possible, and desirable to allow the patient to continue to discharge some of his usual responsibilities from the hospital bed. Today's hospital is decentralizing its decision-making patterns, and this particular change in organizational style would be best served by allowing hospital patients degrees of independence.

Under these circumstances, it seems sensible to suggest that traditional admission practices be brought up to date. It is reassuring to know that some hospitals are moving in this direction. Some hospitals collect most of the information previously collected during the admission interview before the patient comes to the hospital. This practice permits the hospital to admit the patient to the bed without undue delay. The practice of collecting necessary information before the patient comes to the hospital would facilitate an admission procedure that by-passed the delay in the Admission Office. The patient could be taken directly to the hospital "floor," and the remainder of the admission interview could take place after the care of the patient had begun.

When a physician recommends hospitalization, society interprets this to mean that the individual concerned is having a health crisis. Consequently, most patients arrive at the hospital believing that they are the victims of crises. The hospital denies the patient this crisis status unless he is in obvious need of immediate medical attention. Lack of crisis recognition is likely to have one of two possible consequences.

If the patient's sense of personal crisis is strong, he will remain immersed in his own crisis, and he will be relatively unresponsive to all outside influences. Under the impact of a personal crisis, the individual's perception of those things immediate to his situation are exaggerated while his perception of extraneous stimulation is sharply decreased. Thus, a patient who retains a strong sense of personal crisis will be unlikely to remember the information he was given as part of his "welcome to the ward." At some later date, the patient's failure to remember the information that he was given may earn him the reputation of being stupid.

If the patient's sense of personal crisis is weak, he becomes aware of, and is likely to be distressed by, the hospital's refusal to recognize the crisis that precipitated hospitalization. Under this circumstance, the patient's anxiety level increases and anxiety-releasing behavior must be expected. Such patients typically confront refusal to recognize crisis in one of two ways. The patient may try to earn the assurance that help will be available to him when it is most needed by drawing the staff's attention to his limiting his demands for attention. This particular response can be expected from heart and stroke patients. Patients in these diagnostic conditions cannot afford to cry "wolf." Or the patient may draw attention to his situation by making frequent, and relatively trivial, demands on the staff. This response can be expected if the onslaught of a medical crisis is likely to leave the patient in a position to say, "I told you so." Those who work with hospital patients should realize that a sense of personal crisis is inevitably associated with the mere notion of hospitalization.

Hospital patients may experience two different kinds of crisis during the course of hospitalization: the personal crisis and the community crisis. The characteristic response to a personal crisis is quite different from the characteristic response to a community crisis in spite of both the community and the personal crisis producing similar distortions in perception. A community crisis, hurricanes, earthquakes, and the like, triggers what Fritz [2] calls community-of-sufferers behavior. The close supportive relationships among patients frequently found on wards is an example of typical community-of-sufferers behavior. The rapid improvement in working relationships that occur when hospital staff confronts a medical crisis

[2] C. E. Fritz, *Convergence Behavior in Disasters: a Problem in Social Control.* Report prepared for the Committee on Disaster Studies with J. H. Mathewson (Washington, D.C.: National Academy of Sciences, National Research Council, 1957), p. 941. Also C. E. Fritz and H. B. Williams, "The Human Being in Disasters: a Research Perspective," *Ann. Amer. Acad. Polit. Soc. Ser.* 309 (1957): 42–51.

is another example of the characteristic response to a community crisis. A personal crisis, famine or hospitalization, triggers behavior similar to that described in preceding paragraphs. For those interested in learning more about personal crisis behavior, Sorokin's[3] work on famine victims is recommended.

Those who work with patients need to be able to recognize and differentiate these two kinds of behavior because of their strikingly different consequences. Community crisis behavior, the "we're-all-in-the-same-boat" response, increases the patient's sense of social cohesion, and this increase provides psychic support during stress and anxiety. Personal-crisis behavior, the "why-pick-on-me" response, has the opposite consequence. It decreases the patient's sense of social cohesion, and makes him less able to sustain stress. A sense of community crisis has a therapeutic component. A sense of personal crisis increases stress; it does not strengthen the patient's ability to sustain stress.

Although hospital personnel deny crisis status to most hospital patients, they recognize the need to diagnose and treat all conditions labeled "hospital sickness." The usual practice in hospitals is to separate the needs arising from the patient's sickness into a number of separate tasks, and to allocate these tasks to various categories of hospital specialists. Thus, the patient's initial anxiety is decreased because treatments and procedures are being brought to bear on the crisis that precipitated hospitalization. His anxiety tends to be increased, however, because of his lack of familiarity with the hospital situation because of the strangeness of the treatments and procedures to which he is being subjected, and because, having been separated into a number of tasks, he is somewhat puzzled about where he should turn for help and information.

The nurse's role as "tackler-of-tasks" is strikingly evident to the patient, and he tends to turn to her for help and for information. Usually the nurse is able to see to it that the patient's need for help is met, but his need to ask questions frequently places the nurse in a difficult position. In order to defend themselves against these awkwardnesses, nurses tend to establish stylized responses to the patient's requests for information. In the past, it was the fashion to keep the patient uninformed. More recently, it has become the fashion to keep the patient somewhat informed. My observations suggest that both methods have merit. Some patients seem least affected by the stress of hospitalization when they are in a state of blind dependence on omniscient hospital specialists. Others seem to thrive on understanding what is happening to them. Some patients seem to shift from one category to another during the course of a single hospital stay.

These apparently contradictory reactions are the function of differences

[3] P. A. Sorokin, *Man and Society in Calamity* (New York: E. P. Dutton & Co., Inc., 1942).

in personality, class, ethnic background, diagnosis, and temporal focus. Ethnic, class, and personality differences have been well documented,[4] and much has been said in a previous chapter about the patient's need to move along a dependence-independence continuum during the course of a single sickness. Information needs are unique to each patient's background, status, hospital sophistication, disease, and the way in which he interprets his disease. Therefore, it seems sufficient to suggest that all these factors be taken into consideration when the physician, the nurse, and other hospital specialists make decisions about each patient's unique information needs. The influences that temporal focus and its consequences have on the information needs of patients is worth considering in some detail.

The value systems of individuals and of societies can be said to have dominant temporal focuses. When the dominant temporal focus is on the past, hospital sicknesses and other disasters are seen as visited upon the individual by angry gods, spirits, or ancestors. When an individual is focused on the present, causes and consequences are disregarded in favor of immediate gratification and symptom relief. Those who focus on the future, on the other hand, can be expected to show considerable anxiety about the implications and consequences of present situations, to experience little anxiety relief at the removal of a symptom, and to need to plan and to work toward future eventualities.[5]

Individuals and societies tend to have dominant temporal modalities. Middle-class Americans, for example, tend to focus on the future. Subcultures in which a straight-laced deity has made it quite clear what sin is and is not, tend to focus on the possibility that sickness is a punishment for past sins. Those who live at subsistence level in industrial societies tend to focus on the present.

Under the stress of hospitalization, sudden changes in temporal focus should be expected. Cognizance of a particular patient's immediate temporal focus may help the hospital specialist to decide what sort of information the patient needs at any particular moment. To this end, it makes a difference to know whether the patient is appeasing his gods and easing his conscience, whether he is seeking immediate relief and gratification, or whether he is trying to understand the implications of his predicament and struggling to plan for the future. Mobilized guilt suggests past focus; longing for creature comforts present focus. An expressed need for real-

---

[4] Dr. E. L. Brown's treatment of this subject in *Newer Dimensions of Patient Care,* Part 3 (New York: Russell Sage Foundation, 1964) is particularly useful to those who work in hospitals.

[5] An excellent example of this phenomenon is M. Zborowski, "Cultural Components in Responses to Pain" in *Patients, Physicians, and Illness,* 3d ed., E. G. Jaco ed. (New York: The Free Press, 1963), pp. 256–268.

life activities and people suggests future focus. Patients with different temporal focuses may need different items of information under apparently similar situations. Patients with different temporal focuses will use the same item of information in different ways and for different purposes.

Hospitalization tends to decrease the patient's sense of social cohesion by separating him from his natural social environment. Under our present system of centralizing facilities and services into hospitals, the patient is physically removed from the various social groups of which he is a member. However, the various ways in which the hospital dictates the extent of the patient's separation from society can be modified in order to decrease the loss of social cohesion.

Much has been written about the rules and regulations that set limits on visitors. Usual practice excludes children and pets, limits the number of visitors permitted, and dictates the times during which patients may receive visitors. Although visiting regulations have been modified in most hospitals during recent years, they are rarely individualized to an extent that permits the patient to select a "menu" of visitors according to his own needs and preferences. Germs, equal privileges for everyone, and the work of the ward are the reasons most frequently given for not permitting the patient to make decisions about his own visitors. Information obtained from observations and interviews suggest, however, that the nuisance value of visitors often may be the cause that determines the reluctance of hospital management to individualize visiting regulations.

The nurse is the person who most frequently imposes the hospital's regulations for visitors. Observation indicates that nurses are sometimes uneasy during the intrusions of visitors, and that they prefer to be protected by the hospital's regulations from making decisions about patients' visitors. On the other hand, nurses are aware of an individual's expressed need to be visited by persons currently excluded by hospital regulations and sometimes break visiting regulations to the advantage of particular patients. In most cases, these infringments are genuine attempts to meet the pressing needs of particular patients. In a limited number of cases, the evidence suggests that the power to either break or enforce visiting regulations is used as part of an informal reward and punishment system.

It seems sensible to suggest two changes in the management of visiting regulations. One, the development of a systematic approach to visitor orientation as an attempt to reduce the nuisance value of visitors. And two, the establishment of some system of recognizing each patient's need to be visited by one set of persons and protected from another set of persons. Some patients need to be visited by their pets, and it is possible to permit this without disrupting the hospital. I have recorded a number of visits by pets that did not disrupt the unit nor upset those in it.

When a person enters a hospital, society releases him from his usual obligations, and hospital practices tend to restrict his opportunity to discharge these responsibilities. In some cases, a holiday from responsibility is exactly what the patient needs. In other cases, being prevented from discharging real-life responsibilities increases the patient's stress and anxiety. In the latter case, several things may happen. There may be some loss of identity since discharging responsibilities is one way of expressing identity. There may be concern that the group, family, firm, and others, will suffer because the patient is not permitted to discharge his usual group responsibilities. There may be fear that he will lose his place in the group because others will usurp his membership by assimilating his responsibilities during his absence.

The practice of automatically preventing hospital patients from fulfilling their usual responsibilities should give way to a system of decisions based on the needs and capabilities of individual patients. Thus, just as the patient's toileting needs and capabilities are considered when deciding whether he should use the bedpan or be given "bathroom privileges," so a patient's responsibility needs and capabilities should be considered. On the basis of these needs and capabilities, a decision could be made as to whether or not the patient must be relieved of his real-life responsibilities. In some cases, it is therapeutic for the patient to continue to discharge his usual responsibilities.

Temporary membership in the hospital community should compensate, to some extent, for the decrease in social cohesion that inevitably accompanies the patient's separation from society. Unfortunately, hospital roles and practices are ill fitted for this particular function. The traditional patient role is obsolete and recent changes in that role are not yet clearly defined. Orientation to hospital life is inadequate. And the hospital, as a community, seems to the patient to be peopled by a bewildering variety of specialists who never speak to each other. At the present time temporary membership in the hospital community does not contribute to the patient's sense of social cohesion.

8

A Life Line
to Society

As we have seen in previous chapters the traditional patient role is obsolete, and there is considerable pressure to change the role currently imposed on the hospital patient. If we are to modify the patient-role in the direction suggested by contemporary changes in decision-making patterns, we might consider designing these modifications in such a way as to increase rather than decrease the patient's sense of social cohesion. The result would be to decrease the patient's sense of separation from his usual social supports, his relationships with the various social groups of which he is a member. And we could increase the social support available to him from his temporary membership in the hospital community. In order to consciously contrive this sort of increase, we need to understand exactly what our present arrangements tend to do to the hospital patient's sense of social cohesion.

What happens to the sick person who becomes a hospital patient? He prepared himself for this experience by mobilizing social support. When he enters the hospital he is separated, to a greater or lesser degree, from the source of this support. In addition, many of the artifacts that reinforce his identity are removed. During his hospital stay little effort is made to sustain his life line to society although sporadic efforts are made to stir his psyche into supportive action. His temporary membership in the hospital community is a second class affair that rarely manages to increase his sense of belonging to the human race. In this chapter, we will examine the possibility of using the patient-role to maintain the sick person's life line to society. We will use a thesis developed by Durkheim[1] as our organizing principle, and we will translate his concept into suggestions about concrete action.

One of the objects of hospital care is to decrease stress and anxiety. To this end appropriate measures to decrease stress are taken, and attempts are made to increase the patient's ability to sustain anxiety. For the most part, action to support the psyche is based on psychological principles. In an up-to-date hospital, the patient is "psyched out," and a plan of action based on psychological principles is implemented. The possibility of utilizing sociological principles for the most part has been overlooked. Most hospitals inadvertently decrease the patient's psychic strength by depersonalizing him and by restricting his access to support from family, friends, and associates.

Durkheim (1951) in his book *Suicide* presents and supports the thesis that social cohesion provides psychic support to group members during periods of acute stress and anxiety. If we wish to use Durkheim's thesis, we must begin to think about what happens to the sick person's sense of social cohesion when he is hospitalized. When this step has been taken, we can begin to consider various ways in which the nurse and other hospital specialists might capitalize on the hospital experience to increase the patient's sense of social cohesion. If Durkheim is right, this type of action would increase the patient's ability to tolerate the stresses and anxieties inevitably associated with hospitalization.

At the least, hospitalization is a physical crisis for the sick person, and a social crisis for the segment of society to which the sick person belongs. The family, friends, and associates of a sick person who becomes a hospital patient recognize this physical and social crisis by supporting the decision to seek medical help, by increasing the attention paid to the sick person, and by decreasing the demands made on him. These changes increase the patient's sense of social cohesion. It also is true that separation from familiar social and physical surroundings tends to decrease the patient's sense of social cohesion.

When the sick person becomes a hospital patient, the hospital and its specialists take the sick person into custody in order to take jurisdiction over his disease. Many of the ways in which the hospital and its specialists

[1] Emile Durkheim, *Suicide: A Study in Sociology,* trans. J. A. Spaulding, ed. G. Simpson, Introduction by G. Simpson (New York: The Free Press, 1951).

discharge these responsibilities tend to decrease the patient's sense of social cohesion. It also is true that the hospital's willingness to accept the sick person as a patient, and many of the things that are done to and for the patient decrease stress. In short, the hospital and its specialists consciously contrive to decrease patient-stress, while, at the same time, they inadvertently decrease the patient's ability to tolerate stress.

The patient's ability to respond to treatment is decreased by unrelieved anxiety and stress. One of the nurse's primary functions is to relieve anxiety and stress and to prevent the accumulation of unrelieved anxiety and stress. To this end, she institutes supportive measures. The nurse is continually aware that when an additional stress or anxiety is added, it must be balanced out either by direct relief or by increasing the patient's tolerance. For the most part, this nursing intervention is based on sound physiological and psychological principles. It would make the nurse's task of balancing out anxieties and stresses easier if she could introduce a third source of support based on sociological principles.

Although decreasing stress and anxiety is one of the nurse's primary functions, all hospital specialists are aware of the need to decrease stress and anxiety, and they do so whenever it is possible. If all hospital specialists were to add an understanding of the patient's sense of social cohesion to their repertoire of knowledge, attempts to provide psychic support by increasing social cohesion could become extremely effective. A hospital administrator who had acquired considerable understanding in these matters arranged for a dog to become an official visitor to a patient whose single remaining significant relationship was with her dog.

When a sick person becomes a hospital patient, his sense of social cohesion may have been both increased in some ways and decreased in others. Consequently, when the patient is admitted to the hospital bed, the balance between his ability to sustain stress and anxiety and his level of stress and anxiety has been in a state of flux for a measurable period of time. The length of time, and exactly what happened during this period may be extremely useful information to those who care for the patient.

If the patient's ability to sustain stress is not robust under normal circumstances, or if entry to the hospital was abrupt, stress and anxiety levels may be extremely high, and the balancing factors may not be functional. Under these circumstances, we can anticipate the distorted perception of those who are in the acute phase of a crisis. Under the impact of crisis, an individual perceives things immediate to his crisis situation with increased intensity, and things not immediate to that situation with decreased intensity.

The practical implications of the change in perception during the acute phase of even relatively minor crises makes it relevant to describe the nature of that change in this chapter. Imagine that you are sitting on the rim of a well looking at the world around you. Suddenly, you are at the bottom of the well looking at the same world. The world looks completely different. Although the patient does not drop into a well, the same type of dramatic change occurs when a person perceives the world around him during the acute phase of a crisis.

About six years ago, a group of nurses decided to experiment with the way in which they admitted patients to their ward. They experimented with opposite methods: a mechanized method and a personalized method. They hypothesized that the patients who were admitted in a mechanistic manner would not remember enough about the admitting nurse to identify her as frequently as those who were admitted in a personalized manner. Each nurse admitted alternate patients according to these two methods, and a lay person interviewed each patient the day after admission. The results were interesting. As far as the hypothesis was concerned, there was no significant difference between the two groups of patients. Those who had been admitted in a personalized manner did not remember things that identified the nurse more frequently than those who had been admitted in a mechanistic manner. What made an impression on the patient, however, was the admission method. Those who were admitted to the hospital bed in a mechanistic manner talked about being depersonalized and about feeling like inanimate objects, whereas those whose admission was personalized talked about how considerate, understanding, and friendly the nurse whom they could not identify had been. This experiment produced an excellent example of typical crisis perception. It also produced an insight into the difficulty inevitably encountered when the nurse with traditional training attempts to modify the procedures to which she has become accustomed. The personalized admission method called for in the experiment described above included allowing the patient to decide whether or not he wanted to go to bed. Fairly frequently, the patient preferred to remain clothed and to either sit in the room or wander about. Most of the nurses found it extremely difficult to tolerate this particular decision. They felt as if they had "unfinished business on their hands," and they returned to the patient repeatedly to see if he was "alright." The nurse is not the only hospital specialist who finds it difficult to abandon accustomed procedures. Most of those who work in hospitals find it extremely difficult to introduce innovations even when they are intellectually committed to do so. The hospital's stylized way of life does not encourage changes that seem to permit the patient to get "out of hand."

The changes in perception that occur when a person is plunged into a crisis have practical implications for all of those who work with sick people. As far as the hospital patient is concerned, he may be in the acute phase of a crisis when he enters the hospital. He may, however, be plunged into a crisis at any time during the hospital stay. That perception is distorted in a characteristic manner during a crisis, and that experiences which seem to be everyday matters to hospital staff may precipitate a crisis in the patient combine to complicate the process of communicating with patients. Thus, those who work with patients must learn to identify the presence of crisis in their patients for a twofold reason: because it produces distortions in communication and because the unrelieved anxiety and stress that characterize crises decrease the patient's ability to respond to treatment. The hospital's habit of denying the crisis status of the patient is not necessarily therapeutic.

If hospitalization has not been abrupt, the sick person may approach the admission desk with an unusually high sense of social cohesion. He has already been through three phases: a first phase during which stresses and anxieties accumulated to a high level; a second phase when his sense of belonging and being cared about was rapidly increased by family, friends, and associates; and a phase during which the physician diagnosed his health problem, and decided what should be done about it. The transactions in the Admission Office tend to erode his sources of psychic support and to increase his anxiety. Those who work in the Admission Office must secure certain items of information about the patient and about his affairs before they can admit him to the hospital. This process tends to decrease the patient as a person, to make it clear that the patient is being taken into the custody of the hospital, and to make it *seem* as if the hospital is not particularly interested in attending to the sickness that has caused hospitalization. In a twenty-one-step procedure used by one Admission Office, the patient's eventual destination, a bed in the hospital, is not mentioned or even hinted at during the first thirteen steps of the procedure. "Step Fourteen: If patient's code is determined to be private, ask patient for his room preference." If the patient's code does not so determine, the admitting clerk is instructed in step eighteen: "Ask bed-control clerk to secure specified bed."

The procedure in the Admission Office has been used to illustrate the hospital's habit of decreasing the patient's ability to sustain stress and anxiety because it is relatively easy to analyze the depersonalizing potential of this particular procedure. All hospital procedures have this same potential, and all hospital practices tend to whittle down the patient's ability to deal with his own anxieties and stresses. The question is: How can those who work in hospitals not only decrease the depersonalizing potential of institutionalized procedures but also consciously contrive to increase the patient's sense of social cohesion? I will suggest a frame of reference that might be productive.

We will begin by differentiating those factors that tend to decrease the patient's sense of social cohesion from those that have the potential to increase it:

DECREASING FACTORS	INCREASING FACTORS
Hospitalization Tends To Decrease the Patient's Sense of Social Cohesion:	*Measures That Could Be Used To Increase the Patient's Sense of Social Cohesion:*

1. Physically removes patient from the various social groups of which he is a member.

2. Limits access to patient of other members of these groups.

3. Limits patient's ability to discharge group membership responsibilities.

4. Membership in the hospital community offers the patient a limited sense of social cohesion.

1. Physical removal remains necessary *but* the admission procedure could be modified.

2. Criteria for visitors allowed could be *the expressed social needs of the patient* rather than numbers and categories of visitors permitted by a universal hospital regulation. For example: socially insignificant, boring, and threatening visitors could be either excluded or rigorously limited; and significant visitors could be encouraged and included. Most hospitals exclude children below a specified age, and do not recognize the possibility that a sick person's most significant relationship might be a relationship with an animal.

3. The nurse might help the patient to identify his membership responsibilities and sort them into three categories:

   a. Those which have been either discharged or delegated—the patient may need reassurance.

   b. Those which can be discharged from the hospital bed—the patient may need help.

   c. Those which can be delegated to others—the patient may need help.

   d. Areas of a sense of excessive responsibility—the patient may need help and reassurance.

4. A systematic attempt could be made to increase the patient's sense of being a member of the hospital community.

DECREASING FACTORS   INCREASING FACTORS

Hospitalization Tends   *Measures That Could Be Used*
To Decrease the Patient's   *To Increase the Patient's*
Sense of Social Cohesion: *Sense of Social Cohesion:*

a. The treatment and care of patients is organized into the hospital as a number of separate tasks assigned to a number of different specialists and departments.

a. The care and treatment of the patient could be organized into the hospital as three separate but overlapping responsibilities assigned to three people, a nurse, a physician and one administrative person. The single person from administration would handle *all* the hospital's business affairs with the patient. These three people would work together as the patient's basic hospital team.

b. Each staff member or hospital department has discharged his or its responsibility to the hospital as soon as the assigned patient task is completed. The patient may be on the receiving end of transactions with as many as fifty persons in a twenty-four hour period.*

b. The physician, the nurse and the administrative person could be made responsible for all hospital-patient transactions within his or her area of competence. For example: the administrative person would be the only member of the hospital staff with whom the patient or his family would transact business: admission, insurance, billing, discharge, and so forth.

c. Patient participation, as a member of the hospital community, is limited to submitting to the rules and regulations of the hospital and to the decisions of hospital specialists.

c. The patient could participate as a member of the hospital community by becoming an active member of the health team. If his condition permits the patient might, for example, record information concerning those matters about which he alone has first hand knowledge: in and out of bed, eating, eliminating, sleeping, activities, anxieties, and so forth.

* Numerous patients have collected this information for me.

DECREASING FACTORS	INCREASING FACTORS
Hospitalization Tends To Decrease the Patient's Sense of Social Cohesion:	*Measures That Could Be Used To Increase the Patient's Sense of Social Cohesion:*
d. Patients frequently fail to perceive the various categories of hospital specialists as a community. To the patient the hospital community seems fragmented into groups of people who never communicate with each other.	d. If a determined effort were made to refrain from asking the patient the same question over and over again the patient might begin to believe that the hospital is a community of health specialists. He also might believe that he is being cared for by a health team. This could be done in a relatively simple manner. If, for example, the patient is *not* asked questions the answers to which already have been recorded in the chart.

This analysis merely outlines the range of possibilities. It is intended to suggest one way in which those who work in hospitals might begin to think about developing a systematic approach to the problem of creating supportive measures that could stimulate psychic support by increasing the patient's sense of social cohesion. If Durkheim (1951) is right, and there is every reason to believe that he is right, the hospital patient's ability to support stress and anxiety can be increased by increasing his sense of social cohesion. An experimental approach might be developed in the following manner.

The changes in routine ward practices suggested by the analysis above could be a first step toward a systematic use of the hospital's social environment as a therapeutic milieu designed to increase the patient's sense of social cohesion. The changes suggested are simple changes. They merely attempt to arrange matters so that the patient is treated and cared for as a person by people who have acquired the habit of speaking to each other about the patient's problems. These changes in routine practice are interdependent, and combine to form a modified process which differs from routine practice in five particulars. The relationship between the hospital and the patient is simplified. The nurse's responsibility for the patient's social environment is recognized and focused in a nursing tool.[2] The patient is given an active part in recording his own progress. During initial interviews, the patient is not asked a question he already has

[2] Identifying the patient's need to discharge membership responsibilities, to select his own visitors, and so on.

answered in a satisfactory manner. The patient is given a sense of membership in the team of specialists that are caring for him and attempting to cure him. These changes would decrease the depersonalizing potential of task-oriented hospital procedures and increase the possibility of capitalizing on the patient's temporary membership in the hospital community.

This beginning would provide a structure into which other measures to increase the patient's sense of social cohesion could be inserted. It would permit the nurse to collect the information she would need in order to help the patient to feel that he has discharged or delegated his usual responsibilities from his hospital bed in a satisfactory manner. It would also put the nurse in a position to help the patient to implement his own visitor plan. If the patient were to be admitted directly to the ward, as the experimental process suggests, the apparent indifference of the hospital to the patient's disease crisis would be effectively eliminated. The patient and his family would have the additional advantage of dealing with the business side of the hospital as one person rather than as numerous offices dedicated to specialized business tasks.

This change would have a number of advantages. It would permit the patient to become a member of the health team if he wishes to do so, and if his condition permitted. It would encourage the various categories of health specialists to function as a team. It would convince the patient and his family that the hospital is willing and able to diagnose, treat, and care for patients. And it would increase the patient's ability to support stress and anxiety by maintaining his life line to society. In addition, this change is compatible with the hospital's changing decision-making patterns: It decentralizes decision-making to a functional level, the patient.

9

Social Imagination
and the Hospital Patient

In the last three chapters, I looked at the role imposed on hospital patients, suggested that this role was obsolete, and speculated about various ways in which hospitals might modify their expectations of patient behavior. In the preceding chapter, I presented a theoretical frame of reference supporting the notion that successful attempts to increase the patient's sense of social cohesion increases his ability to sustain the stress and anxiety inevitably associated with hospitalization. In this chapter, I present case histories of what I consider successful solutions of the social problems that are encountered over and over again in the hospital. In each case, those who solved the patient's problem used social imagination to do so, and for this reason I have called this chapter "Social Imagination[1] and the Hospital Patient."

[1] I am using the concept of "social imagination" as it is described in C. W. Mills, *The Sociological Imagination* (New York: Oxford University Press, 1959).

THE HOSPITAL STAMP

Mrs. Brown was a "good" patient. She answered when she was questioned, accepted treatment, swallowed pills, and ate what she was given to eat. She did not ask questions, and she made no demands on the staff. Mrs. Brown was fifty-nine years old; she lived with a married son, and she had an unremarkable medical history. Most of those who worked with and for Mrs. Brown considered her a model patient although she did not respond to treatment as vigorously as had originally been expected. The physician was satisfied that Mrs. Brown's lack of resilience was the function of age and a life of hard work. The rest of the staff accepted this opinion. A graduate student in clinical psychology and the nursing student that he was dating were dissatisfied with this explanation. They felt that Mrs. Brown's ability to respond to treatment had been decreased by unrelieved anxiety. They did not mention this contrary opinion to the staff, but they began to concentrate on Mrs. Brown's case.

According to hospital records, Mrs. Brown had been delivered to the hospital by her son. According to the clerk, Mrs. Brown had received no visitors and no letters. No flowers had been delivered to her during her hospital stay. No one had called the hospital to enquire about Mrs. Brown. Mrs. Brown had written one letter, and when the nursing student had asked if she could mail the letter, Mrs. Brown had said: "No, thank you." The staff reported that the letter was kept by Mrs. Brown in her hospital drawer. Mrs. Brown frequently took the letter out of the drawer, and looked at it without taking it out of its envelope. Whenever anyone asked if they could mail the letter, Mrs. Brown said "No, thank you." This evidence suggested that Mrs. Brown was a lonely woman who might fear that her son no longer wished to keep her in his home. The two students had been reading Durkheim's *Suicide,*[2] and they began to think about Mrs. Brown's sense of social cohesion.

Mrs. Brown was allowed to be up and about, but she stayed in bed unless she went to the bathroom or when a staff member asked her to get out of bed. She did not seek conversations with other patients, and when they spoke with her, she replied in monosyllables. When the nursing student asked Mrs. Brown about her family she answered as briefly as possible. It seemed to the two students that Mrs. Brown might be unwanted by her family, not an unusual predicament for the old in our people-scrapping society. They decided that Mrs. Brown's sense of social

[2] Emile Durkheim, *Suicide: A Study in Sociology,* J. A. Spaulding, trans., G. Simpson, ed. Introduction by G. Simpson (New York: The Free Press, 1951).

cohesion could be increased by encouraging her to interact with the other patients. They found that other patients could be encouraged to increase their attempts to interact with Mrs. Brown, but that Mrs. Brown did not accept these invitations.

Mrs. Brown had not brought bedroom slippers with her to the hospital, and the hospital had provided her with their answer to this problem: envelopes of towelling designed to fit large feet. The students noticed that Mrs. Brown seemed to find it difficult to walk in the hospital's slippers. They wondered if Mrs. Brown would be more inclined to socialize if she could move about the ward more easily. The next day the nursing student brought slippers from her dormitory, and "lent" them to Mrs. Brown. Mrs. Brown said: "Thank you." The staff noticed that Mrs. Brown walked about the room when she got out of bed, and during the afternoon, sat in a chair apparently listening while two other patients talked.

That evening the two students had a "study date," but they decided to cut short their time in the library and visit Mrs. Brown. Mrs. Brown was lying in bed looking at her letter. They pulled up chairs, sat down, and said: "Mrs. Brown, we came to visit you because we are worried about you. We know that you are bothered about something, and it bothers us that we can't help you." Mrs. Brown thanked them. She said that everyone was being good to her, and that she was not "bothered."

They looked at Mrs. Brown wondering what to say next. Mrs. Brown lay perfectly still looking at the ceiling. Her letter was lying beside her half hidden by the bedclothes. As the students watched, Mrs. Brown's left hand moved slowly, seeming to search, and came to rest over the letter. Mrs. Brown continued to look at the ceiling. The psychology student suddenly felt that it was important to Mrs. Brown to mail the letter, and he said: "I'll put your letter in the mailbox on my way out of the building." Mrs. Brown looked at the students and said: "Have you got a hospital stamp?" The nursing student said, "Yes, I have a hospital stamp." Mrs. Brown handed her letter to the students, and smiled. She said: "My family has been waiting to hear what happened to me."

Mrs. Brown began to explain. Her son, his wife, and her grandchildren had come with her to the clinic. Her own doctor had told her to bring a suitcase because the hospital doctors might want to keep her. She had left her family in the clinic waiting room, and some hours later was admitted to the hospital bed. She had not seen her family, and she did not know if anyone had told them that the hospital was keeping her. She imagined that her family had waited until the clinic closed, and that they had then returned home. She knew that they would be waiting to hear from the hospital. She had written to them, but she did not have a stamp, and she was not entirely sure that the hospital wanted her to write to her family. The students asked if they could telephone to Mrs. Brown's family. Mrs. Brown said that they did not have a telephone, but she gave the students the telephone number of a neighbor who would call her son or her daughter-in-law to the phone.

Mrs. Brown's family lived about one hundred miles from the hospital, and Mrs. Brown had been in the hospital for almost three weeks. The students called the number that they had been given; and, while the neighbor's husband went to get Mrs. Brown's son, the students listened to the neighbor. Mrs. Brown's family had waited until the cleaners came to clean the clinic. Then they had returned home knowing that the hospital must have decided to keep Mrs. Brown. They had arranged with the neighbors to man the telephone at all times, and to have a member of Mrs. Brown's family available at all times. They met the mailman at their mailbox each day, and had made special arrangements about receiving telegrams at unusual hours. They did not know how or when the hospital would communicate with them. But, they knew that the hospital would instruct them, and they had made arrangements to receive any messages from the hospital without undue delay.

The students talked to Mrs. Brown's son, and he relayed these messages to his wife, his children, and the neighbor's family all of whom were gathered around the telephone to receive the hospital's message. The students told them that Mrs. Brown could be visited at certain times of day. They told them about Mrs. Brown's condition, and what was being done about that condition. They told them about the expected outcome of Mrs. Brown's hospital stay, and said that Mrs. Brown would probably need to spend another two or three weeks in the hospital. Mrs. Brown's family and neighbors sent comforting messages to her, and the students delivered these messages to Mrs. Brown that night.

The following day Mrs. Brown's family visited her in the hospital. Her son's employer had given him the day off, and had sent flowers to Mrs. Brown. Mrs. Brown's neighbor had come with the family, and many messages from community members were delivered. From that moment until Mrs. Brown left the hospital, her life in the hospital was quite different from what it had been while she had lain in bed wondering about how to get a stamp for her letter. Her family visited her at the weekend, and during the week Mrs. Brown "visited" with the other patients on the ward. Mrs. Brown seemed to respond to treatment more vigorously, and she was discharged from the hospital ten days later.

THE SNUFF CHEWER

Mr. Jones was admitted to the hospital with a head injury and a number of stigmas. The physicians and nurses who looked after Mr. Jones cared for him in a competent manner. Before he was discharged from the hospital, they came to realize that the stigmas which he had brought with him had prevented them from giving Mr. Jones the kind of care he needed during part of his hospital stay.

Mr. Jones had injured his head while resisting arrest during a drunken fight, and he was brought to the hospital by the arresting officer. As long as it was uncertain whether Mr. Jones would live or die, his status as a prisoner and the fact that he had been injured while drunk and resisting arrest did not interfere with the ability of hospital specialists to give Mr. Jones the best possible care. As soon as Mr. Jones began to recuperate, however, it became increasingly difficult for the staff to tolerate Mr. Jones's idiosyncrasies.

Mr. Jones's behavior was distasteful, and seemed uncouth to most staff members. Instead of asking for a bedpan in a middle-class manner, Mr. Jones would announce that he was "ready to shit." When he could feed himself, residual clumsinesses exaggerated the differences between acceptable middle-class eating behavior, and the eating behavior that seemed polite to Mr. Jones. Mr. Jones was not a heavy cigarette smoker as were some of those persons who cared for him, but Mr. Jones was a heavy snuff chewer. Snuff chewing in a hospital bed, and snuff chewing before he had recovered normal control of his body led to an inevitable consequence: Mr. Jones soiled his hospital gown and the hospital bed. This mess had to be cleaned up by the hospital staff. When this inevitable consequence had repeated itself a number of times, the staff began to feel that prisoner Jones did not deserve, and obviously did not appreciate, what was being done for him.

One nurse talked to him about getting "fighting drunk" and was distressed at Jones's attitude: Jones seemed proud of his ability to get "fighting drunk," and he boasted about the fighting drinkers that ran in his family. Another staff member raised this issue with Mr. Jones, and Jones began to boast about his prowess when drunk. Someone talked to Mr. Jones's brother about Jones's drinking habits. The brother seemed proud because Mr. Jones was a "chip off the old block," the old block being a grandfather who had killed seven men. The staff become increasingly angry about the extra trouble to which Jones put them, particularly when he soiled himself and the bed while chewing snuff.

One day Mr. Jones went for treatment to another part of the hospital, and a nurse, at the suggestion of one of the physicians and supported by the agreement of other staff members, confiscated prisoner Jones's supply of snuff. Mr. Jones kept his snuff in his hospital drawer, and when he returned from the Physical Therapy Department, he opened his drawer to discover that his snuff had disappeared. Mr. Jones looked into the drawer for several minutes, and then he said: "If only they had told me. I know I mess myself up. If they had told me, I would have been more careful." He closed the drawer and said: "There was no call to take it behind my back."

Unknown to Mr. Jones, the nurse who had confiscated his snuff was passing. She saw and she waited to listen. Perhaps she had wanted to see how prisoner Jones took being "put in his place." Perhaps her presence in the hall at that precise moment was a coincidence. It does not matter why the nurse was there. What does matter is the profound effect the patient's response had on the nurse and on the rest of the staff, including the physician who had made the original suggestion. The patient had accepted the hospital's arbitrary action with dignity and regret. The nurse saw prisoner Jones turn into Mr. Jones, a man with integrity who had seemed somewhat less than a person merely because he came from a different subculture, and after being arrested during an attempt to resist arrest while drunk.

The nurse told me that it was a striking experience. Suddenly clues about Mr. Jones's life-style organized her misinterpretations into understanding. She remembered that the policeman had treated Mr. Jones with deference as someone to be admired rather than despised. She thought about the way in which Mr. Jones and his brother had not boasted about Mr. Jones's prowess when drunk until they were invited to do so. And she suddenly realized that the frontier-town society about which she had read in books, still existed and continued to produce folk heroes like Mr. Jones. She also realized that she, herself, had the potential to be misinterpreted by others in much the same way as she and the rest of the staff had misinterpreted Mr. Jones.

The nurse went to cocktail parties, and she was a heavy smoker. She could have had an accident on the way home from a cocktail party. She could be recuperating from a head injury in a hospital where the physicians and the nurses felt strongly about smoking and drinking. She and other members of the hospital staff might have been stigmatized for behavior that seemed perfectly normal to them. The nurse suddenly saw herself, the physician, and some of the other staff members lying helpless on a row of hospital stretchers. A strange nurse was moving among them looking down into their nicotine-stained nostrils. The strange nurse had an expression of exaggerated disgust on her face.

The staff returned Mr. Jones's snuff. Mr. Jones graciously accepted their apologies. Mr. Jones left the hospital telling the staff to "Look for a deer when the hunting season opens." Some weeks later Mr. Jones drove up to the hospital with a deer draped over the hood of his car.

THE MINISTER'S WIFE

Mrs. Smith, the minister's wife, was five-feet-six-inches tall, and she weighed just over ninety pounds. She had been in the hospital for two weeks, and during those two weeks she had gained three pounds. Mrs. Smith had been subjected to numerous diagnostic procedures, and the physicians had been unable to find a satisfactory explanation of Mrs. Smith's gradual weight loss. Mrs. Smith had been losing weight for two years. A psychiatric consultation had yielded no satisfactory answer to the problem. When the physicians failed to find an answer, the nurses began to wonder whether Mrs. Smith's social situation might be at fault. They decided to "psyche her out," and they began to spend time encouraging Mrs. Smith to talk about herself and about her life situation. There was nothing extraordinary about either Mrs. Smith or her life situation.

Mrs. Smith had been a social worker before her marriage, and she seemed genuinely delighted when her husband and their three children visited her in the hospital. Family reunions were observed by the staff, and the staff talked with and liked Mr. Smith and the three children. These reunions took place in the waiting room because the youngest child, a boy of eight, was too young to enter the ward. Mrs. Smith seemed to enjoy her family, and her accounts of her everyday life suggested that she enjoyed the role of minister's wife. She did say that the youngest child was unplanned, and that she had been disappointed when she discovered that she was pregnant. She had planned to work as a social worker as soon as the second child entered first grade. The family had not had an unusually difficult time, and there had been no tragedies among either friends or relations. They had moved to her husband's present parish two years ago.

The nurses consulted a convenient sociologist who was an expert about family life. In the absence of obvious difficulties in Mrs. Smith's personal life and social situation, they began to look at minor contradictions as possible clues. They found a minor contradiction. Mrs. Smith had wanted to work when her second child had begun first grade, and had been disappointed when she became pregnant. The child who had prevented her from returning to work was finishing second grade, but Mrs. Smith had not become a social worker again. The family-life expert talked to Mrs. Smith about the shortage of trained social workers, and asked her about the jobs available to social workers in the town in which she, Mrs. Smith, lived. Mrs. Smith talked freely and at length. One of the nurses present said: "You certainly wouldn't find it difficult to get an interesting job."

Mrs. Smith said: "I have decided not to get a job until John (the eight-year-old) is older."

Two days later, a comment by the sociologist triggered a conversation that gave the staff the clue they had been looking for. The sociologist and Mrs. Smith were talking about what Mrs. Smith did as a minister's wife. The sociologist said: "I don't think I could be a minister's wife. I couldn't stand bringing children up under the eyes of a whole congregation. I wouldn't like to feel that I had to be hospitable to people that I might not like. And I would hate to attend meetings that I might not be interested in." The minister's wife began to cry.

When she had finished crying, she explained that she had planned to start work when John, the eight-year-old, entered first grade, but that her husband had been moved that same year. She had decided to wait until the family had settled in the new parish, and then get a job. During the first months in the new parish, she began to feel that her husband's new parishioners would object to her working. She had talked to some of them about the possibility, and they had seemed surprised that she would want to work. During the past year, she had felt trapped by her role as minister's wife, and she felt guilty because she had come to resent the necessity of attending meetings merely because she happened to be the minister's wife.

During the next days, the staff talked with Mrs. Smith about the feminine role in our society, and about the working mother who, once a rarity except at low socioeconomic levels, had become an acceptable member at all levels in our society. Before Mrs. Smith left the hospital, she had rehearsed her strategy with her husband's parishioners. She needed no strategy with her husband and their children; they expected her to become a social worker as soon as her health improved. Mrs. Smith began to gain weight rapidly, and to take pains with her grooming. Ten days later, the physicians decided that Mrs. Smith could leave the hospital.

Three months later, Mrs. Smith went to a social work convention, and on her way home she stopped off at the hospital to visit. It was lunch time, and Mrs. Smith decided to look in the cafeteria before she visited the in-patient unit. Two of the nurses she knew were sitting with a third person having lunch. Mrs. Smith pulled up a chair, and began to talk. She obviously knew the two nurses extremely well. And it was equally obvious that they could not place Mrs. Smith.

Mrs. Smith looked like a person whom the nurses might have met at a cocktail party or during a workshop. She was well dressed and slender; she looked well, and she seemed to be delighted with life. After a few minutes, Mrs. Smith realized that the nurses had not recognized her, and she told them who she was. One of the nurses said: "You look so different. I was trying to remember where we had met. It is terrible that I didn't know you." Mrs. Smith said: "It isn't terrible. It is one of the nicest things that has ever happened to me."

MISS DARWIN'S WORKSHOP

Miss Darwin was described on the chart as a sixty-two-year-old, white female. Miss Darwin had been Academic Dean at a well-known college for women. She was particularly knowledgeable about Seventeenth-Century English Literature, and she was interested in seashells. She had been on her way to Sanabelle Island to collect shells when it had become necessary for her to enter the hospital. Miss Darwin did not have "bathroom privileges," and the physician became interested when he discovered that Miss Darwin had wet her bed three days in a row.

The physician was puzzled. The patient's physical condition did not satisfactorily explain these accidents, and these accidents were not at all Miss Darwin's style. The physician talked it over with the nurse. The nurse was somewhat in awe of her distinguished patient, but she enjoyed talking with her, and she had dropped into the habit of visiting Miss Darwin whenever she had a free moment. The nurse began a discrete investigation, and discovered that she, herself, had inadvertently precipitated a subtle attack on Miss Darwin. The attack was intended to irritate and inconvenience the patient. But, Miss Darwin's sense of dignity had turned the attack into an ingenious assault.

The attacker, an aide who was on notice to leave at the end of the month, was getting back at the nurse whom she thought had caused her dismissal. The aide had noticed that the nurse liked and seemed to admire Miss Darwin. The aide decided to attack her enemy, the nurse, through this particular patient whom she thought of as the nurse's "pet." The aide set out to irritate and inconvenience the patient by placing the bedpan out of reach, and by presenting it at her own convenience after it had been asked for. The patient did not seem to the aide to be unduly perturbed, and the aide began to delay her responses to the patient's requests in order to "get a rise" out of her. The inevitable consequence disturbed the patient acutely, and she was not able to conceal this from the aide. The aide had been able to repeat her victory twice before the physician became puzzled, and asked the nurse to investigate. The nurse quickly discovered what had been happening, and the aide left the hospital for good that very day.

Miss Darwin remained in the hospital for another month, and during this month Miss Darwin and the staff engaged each other in a profitable dialogue. The staff had not previously thought that the patient is at the mercy of the hospital's staff. It had not occurred to them that a job in a hospital might be attractive precisely because it provided opportunities to exercise power over other people. During what the staff came to call "Miss Darwin's workship," the practical implications of this particular possibility were examined.

It was obvious that the patient places himself in jeopardy if he reports minor insults and infringements. Miss Darwin and the staff began to work out various ways in which the physician and the nurse could detect such behavior. The aide who had attacked Miss Darwin had drawn attention to her mistreatment of the patient; she could not resist recording the accidents that she had precipitated. She wanted a nurse whom she disliked to think that a valued patient was merely an incontinent, old woman. This aide's action is not typical of the problem.

The mistreatments that the staff began to look for after Miss Darwin's workshop are concealed, and therefore most easily accomplished when there is least supervision. It became obvious that those persons who seek unpopular shifts, and unpleasant tasks that coincidentally remove them from supervision should be watched until they can be trusted not to mistreat patients. Although the patient hesitates to speak out, he may betray his predicament in subtle ways when a third person is present. If the physician and the nurse are alert to this possibility, they notice that the patient sends out silent signals that all is not as it should be. And when the patient leaves the hospital, he may be prepared to speak out if the matter is raised. These practices are now incorporated into the supervision patterns of those who attended "Miss Darwin's workshop," and, although the incidence of untrustworthy staff is extremely low, persons of this type are now detected before they have done considerable damage.

THE BIRTHDAY CAKE

Mrs. Jones was a thin, quiet woman who appeared to be about fifty although she was only thirty-four years old. Mrs. Jones' heart had been severely damaged when she was four years old, and she had led an extremely restricted life. She was in the hospital being evaluated for possible heart repair. Mrs. Jones was a "poor risk," but both she and her husband felt that they wanted to take this slim chance. Mrs. Jones wanted to live before she died, and she was prepared to risk death for the possibility of life. The surgeon agreed to operate in a month's time, and the nurses were planning Mrs. Jones' postoperative care.

As far as the postoperative care of the patient was concerned, the central problem was that Mrs. Jones would not ask anyone for anything however badly she might need it. Mrs. Jones' absolute refusal to ask for help when she needed it would make it almost impossible to provide Mrs. Jones with the care that she would need after her operation. The nurses were determined to find a solution to this problem.

Mr. Jones said that his wife was "like this with everyone except himself," and he could not suggest a solution. The surgeon had no useful suggestions to make, and Mrs. Jones refused to discuss the matter. The nurses decided to look for clues in the meager information that they had about the patient as a person.

The only visible clue was that Mrs. Jones read the Bible incessantly. She ignored all overtures, and she could not be engaged in a conversation even about the Bible. The nurses had noticed that Mrs. Jones seemed to read only one portion of the Bible. They were able to discover unobtrusively that Mrs. Jones read the Book of Job, over and over again. All the nurses read Job. And, because this was their only clue, they attempted to learn something about Mrs. Jones by thinking about what Job's story might mean to Mrs. Jones. The day Mrs. Jones was ready to leave the hospital, a new clue was laid down.

Mrs. Jones was scheduled to be readmitted to the hospital on her birthday. One of the nurses asked Mrs. Jones if she had drawn this coincidence to the surgeon's attention. Mrs. Jones said: "No." The nurse told Mrs. Jones that her admission could be rescheduled if she wished to spend her birthday at home. For the first time since she had been admitted to the hospital, Mrs. Jones began to talk to someone other than her husband. She explained that when she was a child, her family had been very poor, and that she and each of her six brothers and sisters had celebrated their birthdays by having a favorite cake baked. Her birthday cake had been an orange cake.

Mrs. Jones' mother lived forty miles from the Jones' home, and each year Mr. Jones drove his wife to her mother's home on Mrs. Jones' birthday so that she could eat a slice of the orange cake that her mother had baked for her. The previous year Mrs. Jones' mother had forgotten her daughter's birthday. When the Jones' had arrived, there was no orange cake. Mrs. Jones had decided that this year she would use the energy it took to be driven forty miles to bake an orange cake for herself. She said: "I might just as well be in the hospital as baking a cake."

The nurses decided that they would see to it that Mrs. Jones had an orange cake for her birthday. This decision was not a mere sentimental gesture. An orange cake was much more than a cake to Mrs. Jones. The nurses hoped that if the hospital recognized Mrs. Jones' birthday with an orange cake, Mrs. Jones might permit the hospital and its specialists to take her mother's place, and care for her. They hoped that the cake would make it possible for Mrs. Jones to ask for help when she needed it.

They were right. Mrs. Jones returned to the hospital on her birthday. After dinner that evening, the orange cake was brought into the room. Mrs. Jones ceremoniously cut her cake, took the first slice, and insisted that a slice be cut for the other patient in the room and for each member of the nursing staff. A large slice was cut and set aside for the surgeon.

Mrs. Jones rested in the hospital for two weeks before her operation, and the staff was confident that they would be able to give Mrs. Jones the best possible care after her operation. She no longer hesitated to ask when she needed something. She talked with the staff and with other patients. She continued to read her Bible, but she sampled around in it; she did not continuously read Job. She asked her husband to buy her a new nightgown; he bought three. She spent time fixing her hair, and she began to use lipstick.

Mrs. Jones never returned from the operating room, and it took the staff some time to realize that they had succeeded in giving Mrs. Jones superb care. Mr. Jones told me that before she died, his wife had told him to tell the nurses that the two weeks in the hospital before her operation had been "two of the happiest weeks in her life." The staff had not saved Mrs. Jones' life, but they had brought her back into life before she died.

Many hospital procedures contain reminders that the patient is a person, but the human problems that are collected in the hospital would go undetected and remain unsolved unless those who work in hospitals not only cared for patients but also cared about them. In this chapter, I presented the heart of the matter, human problems, and successful attempts to solve them. In the final chapters of *In Horizontal Orbit,* we will look briefly at the relationship between professional health workers and at their relationships with the patient. We will begin with these relationships in the hospital, and then speculate about what happens when these relationships leave the hospital and enter the community.

10

That Fascinating Triangle.
Physician, Patient, Nurse

If the changes suggested in previous chapters were to become routine practice, the patient's role and his relationships with the physician, the nurse, and with other members of the health team would be modified. In order to identify the modifications that would become necessary, we must examine existing roles and relationships. It will be simpler to do so if we limit ourselves to that fascinating triangle: the physician, the nurse, and the patient. These three persons occupy what we might think of as the basic roles in what now is thought of as the health team. Let us examine the way in which these three persons approach each other and begin to establish a relationship.

The patient seeks cure; as we have seen, he approaches the physician. The physician scrupulously avoids making the first move, and he uses considerable ritual during the process of receiving the patient, diagnosing his condition, and deciding on a course of treatment. Unless there is an acute crisis that demands immediate attention the patient enters an outer office, establishes his right to be there, and is told to wait until the physician is ready to receive him. When in due course his turn comes, he is summoned by a nurse with a chart in her hand who proceeds to prepare him for the physician. She collects information about such things as his weight, temperature, pulse rate, and blood pressure; and she may collect samples of blood, urine, and sputum from him. She installs him in an examining room either on a chair or on the examining table, and in some cases she sees to it that he removes his clothes, and puts on an examining robe. If the patient's physical crisis is not severe, and if he is familiar with the treatment he is about to receive, this part of the approach ritual has amusing overtones as the following account by a woman who had arranged to have the wax washed out of her ears suggests.

> The nurse led me to the scales. I said: "I don't need to be weighed; I'm here to have my ears washed out." She said: "Doctor likes to get vital signs on all patients." The nurse led me to a room, and asked me to sit on the end of the table. She took my temperature, pulse, and blood pressure, and when these had been recorded, she asked me to lower my dress to my waist, and I said: "I don't need to undress, he's going to wash out my ears." She said: "Doctor wants all patients prepared in this way." After I had lowered my dress, she refastened the blood pressure cuff around my arm. While she was doing so, I said: "You don't need to take it again, for heaven's sake. My blood pressure does not go up when I strip to the waist." She said: "Doctor wants all patients cuffed in case he wants to take their blood pressure."

The patient waits in the examining room for a considerable period of time. Eventually, the physician enters, looks at the chart, greets the patient, and begins to examine him. In most cases, it is obvious to the patient that the physician has examined him thoroughly, and has given considerable thought to the problem before he delivers a diagnosis. He names the problem, he tells the patient what the label attached to his complaint means in terms of change in condition and consequences, and he prescribes a course of treatment. The patient is then dismissed by the physician who enters another examining room, leaving the patient to find his own way out.

Space, time, and the way in which the patient is prepared for the physician combine to establish social distance between them. In most cases this distance is reinforced by the transaction between physician and patient in the examining room. The patient seeks cure, and he is assisted during his approach to the physician by the nurse who approaches him, and does whatever she and the physician have decided must be done before patients are examined. Both in the physician's office and in the hospital, the nurse approaches the patient, and does whatever needs to be done to and for him. In the hospital the nurse remains close to the patient, whereas the physician looks in on his patient. The nurse comes when the patient asks for care, and she comes to give him care when she knows that he needs it. The nurse's use of time and space, and that she approaches the patient even when he does not ask her to do so reduce the social distance that separates the patient from the nurse. When we examine the social distance that separates the patient from other members of the health team, we find that the social distance established by each specialty between its members and the patient are similar to those established either by the physician or the nurse.

If we look at what each specialty does, we can see that it is an elaborated version of something once done either by the nurse or the physician. The dietitian, the social worker, the occupational therapist, and the physical therapist have elaborated and specialized services, previously provided by the nurse. They do not approach the patient until they have been requested to do so by the physician, but during their encounters with the patient they tend to reduce the social distance between themselves and the patient in much the same way as the nurse does. As each nurse-derived speciality becomes more sophisticated, its members tend to increase the social distance between themselves and their patients. This tendency is most marked, at least as far as my own observations are concerned, in the psychiatric social worker, who seems to increase social distance by insisting that the patient cannot be helped unless he either asks to be helped or admits that he needs it, and is willing to accept it. In short, the patient is expected to approach and place the problem under the jurisdiction of the therapist in much the same way as he approaches the physician. As we have seen, to do so increases social distance. Physician-derived specialities, radiology, for example, retain the social distance that characterizes the relationship between the physician and his patient, and they establish and reinforce it in a similar manner. Thus, although a cumbersome health technology has produced a large number of differently specialized persons, the relationship of the patient to all members of the health team is similar to his relationship either with the physician or with the nurse. These three relationships can be diagramed as shown in Figure 5.

The proliferation of specialities has affected, to a greater or lesser extent, the decision-making rights of the physician, the nurse, and the patient. The physician has been least affected; his decision-making rights remain clear cut. He remains responsible for diagnosis and treatment, and although he may turn to other specialities for assistance, he makes final decisions about what diagnostic procedures will be used, he names the disease, and he decides what should be done about it. Until the patient enters a hospital, his decision-making rights remain more or less intact. If the patient has a condition that is considered dangerous to others, he can be coerced into satisfactory action: The decision-making rights of a person with a contagious disease are limited in this way. If he has a

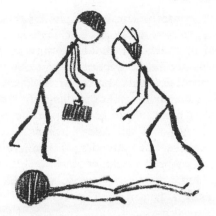

Figure 5. The distribution of decision-making rights and the social distances that characterize the basic triad in the health team.

condition that endangers himself but is not a direct threat to others, he is left more or less free to decide what he is prepared to do about it. There are, of course, social pressures similar to those described in a previous chapter which do not leave him as free to make decisions about his health as he may imagine he is. In a sense there are two sick-roles. A policed sick-role that society imposes when it must protect itself as well as see to it that the sick person is cared for, and a catered-to sick-role in which society decreases the demands made on the sick person, and grants him special privileges as long as he, the sick person, shows that he wants to get well. When sick persons enter a hospital, the difference between these two sick-roles is obscured by the institutionalized role of the hospital patient. It is not easy to differentiate between the two sick-roles in a hospital setting because the decision-making rights of all hospital patients are limited, and the sick person who was catered-to before he came to the hospital tends to be policed when he is in it. The nurse's decision-making rights have been obscured, and as a consequence her function is not clearly understood by other members of the health team, and her relationships with them tend to be ambiguous. A number of causes have contributed to this state of affairs, but the primary one is that the nurse expresses her role by assuming different functions during different shifts. She pinch-hits for other members of the health team if they are absent when the patient needs them. Every other specialized person on the health team has clearly delineated functions that remain stable around the clock.

The changes suggested in the last chapter would provide opportunities for the patient to become an active member of the health team. This increase in function would be therapeutically advantageous, and it would help to differentiate the two sick-roles. The person in the catered-to sick-role would be able to speak out about the way in which the rules and regulations of the institution are applied to him. An opportunity to make choices whenever possible would automatically decrease the appearance of what could be mistaken for police action. The person in the policed sick-role, on the other hand, would be in a position to choose one of two roles: a self-policed role or a sick-role in which he is policed by others. It is reasonable to suppose that providing the patient with an opportunity of choosing to be self-policed would decrease our reluctance to recognize that all societies, including our own, impose a policed sick-role when they consider the sick person dangerous. The treatment previously meted out to the leper is a classical example.

In our society the sick person and those close to him retain the right to decide to seek medical help unless society considers the sick person's condition a threat to others. Under the latter circumstance, society acts to protect itself. Once the sick person has been institutionalized, however, the traditional patient role is imposed on him. This role tends to expose those in the catered-to sick-role to being treated as if they were in the policed sick-role. If all patients in both sick roles were given opportunities to become members of the health team, misplaced police action would disappear and four patient roles would emerge.

The person in the catered-to sick-role would be able to choose between the two roles described in a previous chapter. The experiment mentioned in that chapter permitted the patient to choose between a dependent role and a cooperative role, and it allowed him to change roles when he found it necessary to do so. The changes suggested in the previous chapter would formalize the opportunity to make such a decision. The person whose condition made it necessary to place him in the policed sick-role could choose either to cooperate with the health team, and police himself or he could refuse to take this responsibility, and be policed by others. If the policed sick-role were to be differentiated in this manner, it would be profitable to reexamine the conditions that currently qualify persons for the policed sick-role. Two categories of pathology qualify persons from all socioeconomic levels in our society for the policed sick-role: communicable diseases and gross psychic disturbances. In addition, any lower socioeconomic person who is considered sick enough to need medical help, whether or not he is able to pay for it, automatically assigned to the policed sick-role although those who work in hospitals are not always aware of their tendency to be more arbitrary with an indigent patient than they are with other patients. The serious diseases for which indigent patients are hospitalized include normal childbirth. The qualifications for the policed sick-role might be reexamined.

The development of a second welfare structure which has emerged as a consequence of our War on Poverty[1] gives notice that it is no longer considered profitable to attempt to impose prepackaged solutions to problems on any person in our society, including those at lower socioeconomic levels. It seems reasonable to assume, therefore, that our traditional approach to the health problems of the poor have become obsolete. If this is true, mere indigency should cease to qualify a sick person for the policed sick-role. Society seems to be suggesting that all patients, irrespective of their ability to pay, should be automatically admitted to the catered-to sick-role unless their *diseases* make it necessary to assign them to the policed sick-role.

It will not be as easy as it might seem to make this particular change. All humans are culturally conditioned creatures, and tend to distrust and to stigmatize those who have been conditioned to alien cultural patterns. It will be difficult for the professional health worker to resist imposing prepackaged help on those whose attitudes and behavior are alien and, as a consequence, seem wrong. We expect to encounter alien behavior when we attempt to help foreigners, but we tend to assume that all Americans have the same attitudes and behavior patterns as our own. This tendency will make it difficult to automatically assign the indigent patient to the catered-to sick-role. The indigent patient frequently comes from a subculture that seems alien to the health specialist. One solution would be to increase the health specialist's understanding of the various subcultures in our society. An introduction to this kind of information is presented in a later chapter.

Psychic disorders, particularly when the behavior produced by the disorder seems threatening, ensures assignment to the policed sick-role. Our traditional fear of the insane has abated since the turn of the century, but there is a residual tendency to stigmatize the mental patient. In some segments of our society, it has become fashionable to boast about one's analyst. Even among these populations, however, the need to hospitalize the patient with psychic disorders creates social awkwardnesses which suggest that some stigma is still attached to mental illness. At the other extreme, there are segments of our society in which attitudes about those with psychic disorders remain unchanged. Consequently different, and in some cases conflicting, attitudes about mental illness are to be found among those who work with sick people. Both the psychiatric patient and the patient for whom a psychiatric consultation has been ordered tend to be shifted into the policed role from time to time and at short notice. In this respect, it is interesting to observe the changes in behavior that occur in an elevator when a person who cannot be readily identified as a staff

[1] An interesting discussion of this phenomenon is presented by B. Davies, "The Jolt to U.S. Social Work," *New Society* (May 25, 1967).

member presses the button for the floor on which the psychiatric unit is located. This change is marked when it is known that the patients from that unit sometimes are encountered on hospital elevators.

Childbirth qualifies the patient for the policed sick-role. At first glance childbirth in those who can afford to have children does not seem to place the patient in the policed sick-role. However, when one carefully examines the attitudes and practices in the prenatal clinic, the delivery room, the nursery, and the postpartum area, one begins to realize that the role assigned to the childbearing woman tends to be policed even when she can afford to pay her hospital bill. In our society childbirth mortality was recognized as a threat to society at the beginning of the present century. As a consequence, pregnancy and childbirth are handled in an arbitrary manner for the supposed benefit of both the mother and her child. Infringements by the patient[2] have the potential to damage the child, and for this reason the patient is more severely reprimanded than would be the case if she had another disease. This attitude tends to permeate the practices on the obstetric unit. One new mother's response was to say: "Having a baby in a hospital is like taking a short course. If you pass the course, the baby is given to you as if you were being awarded a certificate." Another said: "They (the hospital staff) act as if my baby belongs to them." Recent questioning of the therapeutic wisdom of separating mothers from their infants is tending to make the patient-role imposed during childbirth less arbitrary.

Psychic disorders are the most subtle passport to the policed sick-role, and the person who is assigned to this role for this reason tends to serve a life sentence. When these disorders produce threatening behavior, society needs to be protected. When the resultant behavior seems bizarre, others are threatened by its strangeness and feel that they need to be protected. Once the label has been attached, the individual concerned is under suspicion even after he has been "cured." As far as the former patient is concerned, forgetfulness, lack of tolerance, anger, and mere mood change continue to disquiet others even when these manifestations were considered normal prior to hospitalization. The discharged psychiatric patient's behavior must be supernormal. It is interesting to speculate about the idiosyncrasies which would have to be erased from one's own behavior patterns if one were to become a "former mental patient."

A communicable disease is the least subtle passport to the policed sick-role. The threat to others is visible, and the precautions that must be taken are both necessary and straightforward. Social considerations complicate our attitudes about some communicable diseases, but these complicating factors are relatively easy to detect, understand, and rectify. Venereal diseases are an excellent example. The policed sick-role might

---

[2] The mother is the patient. It is usual hospital practice *not* to count the infants in the newborn nursery in the hospital census.

well be reserved for those with communicable diseases and gross psychic malfunction. If this limit were set, two advantages would accrue. We would eliminate our reluctance to recognize a need for the policed sick-role; and it would be relatively easy to establish two different sick-roles. In our society we protect others from communicable diseases, and we attempt to cure those with communicable diseases. As far as communicable diseases are concerned, we have nothing to feel guilty about when we impose a policed sick-role. The same lack of guilt would accompany the necessary limits placed on psychiatric patients.

If the patient is either unwilling or unable to participate in the policing process, the health team *must* take appropriate action. When the patient is both willing and able to participate the opportunity to do so would act as an additional guarantee that the necessary precautions were being taken. In this case, the patient would exchange the sense of being policed for the sense of policing himself: An exchange that would be therapeutic for those who are prepared to make it.

Would it be possible for the physician, the nurse, and other members of the health team to function in relationship to four different patient-roles? The experiment mentioned in an earlier chapter suggests that splitting the catered-to sick-role into two roles, one dependent and the other coopera-tive, presented no insurmountable problem. Bringing the policed sick-role out into the open and splitting it into a policed role and a self-policing role has obvious advantages that might make the health specialist's tasks simpler rather than more complex. The health specialist's primary function, organizing to confront the problems created by sickness, might be sim-plified if the two traditional sick-roles were split, and if each patient were permitted to select either a cooperative or a directed role.

How would four patient roles change the relationship between the two other members of our basic triad, the physician and the nurse? My gen-eralized impression of the nurse-physician relationship is that it is a parallel relationship.[3] The physician sees his patient and writes his orders; he may, or he may not, speak directly to the nurse. For her part the nurse cares for the patient, carries out the physician's orders, and discharges her responsibilities to the hospital. She approaches the physician under two circumstances: When the patient needs something for which an order must be written, and when the physician's medication order seems to be in error. I have asked some hundreds of nurses to describe their best working relationships with physicians, and most of these descriptions could be summed up by the conclusion of one perceptive nurse. She said: "I suppose it isn't a relationship. It is like the parallel play of young children. As long as he (the surgeon) doesn't interfere with what I want to do, I consider it a good working relationship."

[3] It has been my observation that all hospital specialists tend to establish this kind of working relationship with those in specialities other than their own.

What has produced this kind of "good" working relationship? It seems to me that this relationship began during the Great Depression when both the nurse and patient-care were institutionalized. The relationship between the physician and the patient has remained functional primarily because patient-physician relationships are established before the patient enters the hospital, and continue after the patient leaves the hospital. The physician-patient relationship is institutionalized for brief periods only, and these periods of temporary intensification seem to strengthen the relationship. The nurse-physician relationship and the physician's relationship with other categories of hospital specialists, tend to be bred in the institution and to have no life outside of the institution. Under these circumstances, the primary relationship of those employed by the hospital is with the institution that has employed them to render certain specified services to its patient-population.

As far as the nurse-physician relationship is concerned at least one of the institution's expectations strains the relationship between them. The institution expects the nurse to act as a curb on the physician's use of its resources. This expectation places the nurse in an invidious position. The physician has the right to make decisions about the diagnosis and the treatment of his patients. These decisions cannot be implemented unless hospital resources are used. The nurse cannot control the physician's use of these resources unless she challenges his medical decisions, and the nurse cannot openly challenge medical decisions. As a consequence, the nurse who attempts to carry out this particular institutional expectation must do so in an indirect manner by informing on the physician and by making it difficult for him to obtain the supplies that he needs. This behavior is unthinkable to most nurses, and they tend to evade this particular institutional expectation. The expectation is present, however, and it creates awkwardnesses that are not conducive to the development of working relationships.

Many of those who work in hospitals, including the administrator, physicians, and nurses, will question the statement made in the last paragraph. The fact that the institution expects the nurse to police the physician is implicit rather than explicit. The nurse is not *told* that it is part of her job to "ride herd" on the physician, *but* nursing is blamed when floor supplies, dressing, drugs, and so forth, are used extravagantly; nurses are encouraged to make it difficult for physicians to gain free access to these supplies; and information about the extravagances of individual physicians is welcomed. In addition, the floor supplies that are used by the physicians, and according to their directions, are traditionally budgeted as nursing costs. When a lay person directly responsible to hospital administration is put in charge of the management of the patient-care unit, the nurse ceases to be responsible for curbing the physician's use of hospital resources, and one impediment to a productive relationship between the nurse and the physician has been removed.

There is another impeding factor. The relationship between the nurse's right to make decisions and the physician's right to make decisions has not been clearly defined. A functional approach to this problem enables us to see that the responsibilities of the nurse and the physician overlap. An examination of these overlapping responsibilities suggests that an interdependent decision-making system is needed. The physician has two primary responsibilities. He must decide what is wrong with the patient, and he must decide what is to be done about this malfunction. The nurse has three primary responsibilities. She must implement the physician's treatment plan, she must keep the physician appraised of changes in the patient's condition, and she must supplement and facilitate the patient's ability to cope. Under these circumstances parallel decision-making systems are not functional, and it is obvious that an interdependent decision-making system must be established.

The decision-making system that is used by a commander and his staff officer is an example of an interdependent decision-making system.[4] In this kind of system, the commander has primary decision-making rights. He makes final decisions about the battle and about other action to be taken. The staff officer has secondary decision-making rights. He decides what information is crucial to the commander's decisions and supplies it. The nurse and the physician need a somewhat similar decision-making system, but in their case the development of such a system is complicated by the physician and the nurse both having primary and secondary decision-making rights. In short, they take turns as commanding officer. The physician is in command of diagnosis and treatment. The nurse is in command when it comes to supplementing and facilitating the patient's ability to cope. And in both cases, the one in temporary command is dependent on the other for information which is crucial to the decisions that are made.

In all situations where two differently specialized people must work closely together, parallel decision-making systems cease to be functional when they impede the flow of crucial information. Parallel systems solicit information from each other, and volunteered information tends to be taken as an interference. The nurse records vital signs because the physician has solicited this information, but she tends to withhold categories of information that are not routinely solicited. In some cases these items of information are pertinent to the physician's decisions, but they are not volunteered because it might seem as if the nurse were interfering with the physician's right to make decisions. The physician withholds infor-

[4] Observations 1945–1946.

mation which is crucial to the decisions that the nurse is making, but in his case reluctance to interfere with the nurse's right to make decisions is not the usual reason for doing so. Physicians frequently do not understand the nurse's supportive function; and until this matter is clarified, the physician cannot be expected to know what items of information are crucial to the nurse's decisions.

The nurse's supportive function is to supplement and facilitate the patient's ability to cope. When supportive measures were primarily based on physiological principles, the physician was able to recognize what the nurse was doing. He valued her contribution to his patient's welfare, and he was able to provide pertinent information. When the nurse began to use supportive measures that were based on psychological principles, the physician frequently failed to understand what was happening. The nurse's attempts to explain tended to lead physicians to the conclusion that the nurse was neglecting the patient's physical well-being in order to "fool around with half-baked notions that had no practical implications."

Under these circumstances the flow of vital information between the nurse and the physician tends to decrease drastically. The physician ceases to value the nurse's opinion, and he begins to feel that she will not use the information he supplies unless she is forced to do so. The nurse comes to equally unflattering conclusions about the physician, and she tends to adopt the attitude that if the physician wants to know "he can find out for himself." When things have come to this pass, the nurse and the physician avoid each other, and their communication tends to be restricted to the information that is recorded in the patient's chart. Some nurses believe that it is part of their function to protect the patient from the physician. This belief runs counter to most patient's experiences with physicians. Patients sometimes find it difficult to confront the physician, but they rarely feel that they need to be protected from him. I suspect that the nurse's failure to make the physician understand how nurses use psychological principles may have given rise to this notion. The physician may be perfectly competent from a medical point of view, but as far as the nurse is concerned, his failure to understand the significance of psychological factors has demonstrated his incompetence to deal with the patient as a person. This conclusion is not necessarily valid.

This limited communication is not uncommon, and, in contrast, the parallel working relationship described by hundreds of nurses as a "good" relationship is, indeed, good. But it is not good enough. The physician needs to be assured that the nurse uses a system of priorities which do not permit her to let the patient bleed to death while she is nursing his psyche. The nurse needs the physician to recognize and value her unique contribution to patient-care. When mutual trust, respect, and understanding are established, productive nurse-physician relationships emerge.

During the course of the past ten years I have examined a number of nurse-physician relationships which were based on mutual trust, respect, and understanding. In each case an interdependent decision-making system had been developed. The nurse felt free to volunteer information that might prove pertinent to the physician's decisions about diagnosis and treatment. The physician welcomed the nurse's suggestions. In addition, the physician recognized and valued the nurse's unique capabilities, and although he might not always understand her rationale for action, he respected it and valued its results. In each case the nurse and the physician enjoyed working with each other, and the patients for whom they were jointly responsible seemed to prosper.

Although we limited our examination of the relationships of the various members of the health team to its basic triad, the physician, the nurse, and the patient, the points made apply to other members of the team. The hospital expects all its employees to safeguard its resources. It expects them to "ride herd" not only on the physician but also on each other. For example, the Diet Kitchen produces a universally attractive commodity—food—and its employees sometimes suspect that those who work on the wards demand food for the patients in order to eat it themselves. Suspicion tends to create a barrier to mutual understanding, and this lack is further compounded by the decrease in communication that inevitably ensues.

It would be inaccurate to assume that the hospital cannot produce mutual understanding and trust. Its organizational system produces understanding and trust in all parts of the hospital under certain circumstances. Some specialized health teams have developed formal mechanisms to promote mutual understanding. In some cases, an overriding mutual interest produces mutual understanding and trust. And there is one circumstance that produces the ability to function that is usually based on mutual trust and understanding. The hospital and the army are organized to fight battles that rarely break out. During a crisis the hospital, like the army, dramatically increases its ability to function effectively. These crises breed mutual understanding. Some specialities, psychiatry is the most striking example, formally assemble the entire health team at regular intervals. These meetings permit the variously specialized health workers to plan together how available resources will be used to meet the needs of the patients. In other cases, mutual interests override the communication barrier; those who work with children share a common interest, and frequently find it easier to communicate with each other than they do with those members of their own profession who are focused in a different direction.

Assembling a group of differently specialized people, and assigning them to work within the same room on the problems of the same patient-population does not necessarily produce a health team. A team is nurtured by communication. It expresses itself in mutually supportive action. And it is characterized by mutual trust and understanding. When the hospital is organized to encourage mutual understanding, health teams develop and prosper. When the institution is organized, even though quite unintentionally in a way that encourages mutual suspicion, health teams either disintegrate or they fail to materialize.

11

Public-Sector Relationships

The literature about interpersonal relationships does not clearly differentiate public-sector relationships from private-sector relationships, and private sector models tend to be used when public-sector relationships are analyzed. In this chapter, I will use Georg Simmel's[1] analysis of the trader-closed group relationship as a model for one public-sector relationship, the therapist-client relationship. I have selected this model because the trader, like the professional health worker, provides a service. I will use the nurse's relationship with a patient-population to demonstrate how Simmel's analysis of the trader-closed group relationship can be used as an analytic model to clarify the relationship between the professional health worker and his client or patient.

The relationship between the nurse and her patient sometimes is thought

[1] For further elaboration of Simmel's theories, *see* G. Simmel, *The Sociology of Georg Simmel*, K. M. Wolff trans. and ed. (New York: The Free Press, 1950), pp. 402–406.

of as similar to the mother-child relationship.[2] This particular approach has provided insights into the dependent status of the patient. The mother-child model does have disadvantages, however, and attempts to clarify certain aspects of the nurse-patient relationship are frustrated by significant differences between a mother-child relationship and a nurse-patient relationship.

The three most significant differences between the two relationships are differences in temporal focus, differences in direction of involvement, and differences in social distances. The mother-child relationship is a permanent relationship with a past, a present, and a future, whereas the nurse-patient relationship is temporary and focused in the immediate present. The direction of involvement in the mother-child relationship is toward the opposite participant in the socialization process, whereas involvement in the nurse-patient relationship is with those qualities imported into the relationship by the nurse: nursing acts needed, offered, and received. The social distances characteristic of the mother-child relationship have their origin in the child's need to establish a separate identity within a permanent relationship, whereas the nurse-patient relationship is characterized by the abrupt shifts in social distance demanded by the patient.

Identification of the differences between a mother-child relationship and a nurse-patient relationship suggest that we need an analytic model for the nurse's role that contains three primary characteristics: product facilitation; relational mobility; and the ability to tolerate abrupt shifts in social distance. The nurse's role is product-facilitating inasmuch as the relationship between the nurse and her patient-population is expressed in those qualities imported into the relationship by the nurse, namely nursing action. The nurse's role demands exceptional relational ability inasmuch as the nurse is required to maintain a continually changing constellation of instant and temporary relationships. The nurse's role is characterized by a unique combination of extreme remoteness and extreme nearness, capable of changing abruptly from one extreme to the other in response to the immediate demands of individual patients. This particular combination of primary characteristics suggests that the analytic model we seek is a public-sector, as distinct from a private-sector model.

Industrial man has successfully separated organized social life into two parts. The private world of family, friends, and other social groupings organized on an individualized basis; and the public world of large-scale, specialized institutions organized to permit the rapid substitution of one individual for another. Industrial man has not been uniformly successful,

---

[2] An excellent example of the insights produced when this model is used is S. Shulman, "Basic Functional Roles in Nursing: Mother Surrogate and Healer" in *Patients, Physicians, and Illness,* 3d ed., E. G. Jaco ed. (New York: The Free Press, 1963), pp. 528–537.

however, in identifying and implementing the social distances that permit him to function equally effectively in these two entirely different social environments.

Private-sector relationships, those between relatives and friends, are potentially permanent and the social distances established by social usage in the private-sector function to prevent extremes that cannot be sustained and tolerated in a network of permanent cooperative relationships. Private-sector social systems recruit new members by two relatively slow processes: birth and the development of casual acquaintanceships into potentially permanent relationships. The usual methods of ceasing to be a member of a private-sector social system are gradual even in cases of sudden death. The dead member, like the geographically distant member, lingers, as a social entity, long after physical separation. All private-sector relationships are characterized by slowly shifting social distances, potential permanence, and involvement with the opposite participant as an individual.

Public-sector relationships, those between colleagues and with specialists or clients, are potentially temporary. The social distances established by public-sector usages function to permit rapid separation and recruitment, and to promote periodic cooperation. Public-sector social systems recruit two categories of members: producers and consumers. Producer members are selected for their ability to function in vacant specialized slots; and consumer members are recruited by their need for particular goods or services. The usual methods of ceasing to be a member of a public-sector social system are abrupt. Individual producers and individual consumers are replaced rapidly. Permanent slots are reoccupied as soon as they are vacated, and departed members abruptly cease to exist as entities in the institution's social system. All public-sector relationships are characterized by abrupt changes from extreme remoteness to extreme nearness, potential temporariness, and the qualities imported into the relationship of both producer and consumer.

In public-sector relationships, the face-to-face relationship between producer and consumer are modifications of the relationship between the trader and his customer. The trader's role probably began to emerge in Neolithic times; during the Urban period, the trader's role was well established; and the Industrial Revolution forced further modifications of the trader's role. The nurse's role is a public-sector role, and as such is a modification of the classical trader's role. Simmel, a French sociologist who died in 1918, analyzed the trader's role in a brilliant manner. His analysis is available to us from Wolff's translation (Simmel 1950: 402–406).

Simmel's analysis of the trader and his relationships enables us to increase our understanding of the relationship between the nurse and her patient-population. Simmel's description of the trader's relationship to his client group is strikingly similar to the observed relationship between the nurse and her patient-population. The trader's position in his client group is determined by the fact that he has not belonged to it from the beginning, and that he imports qualities into it, which do not and cannot stem from the group itself. It is this unique position in the group that gives the trader's relationship with the group and with individual group members its distinctive character. The trader is at one and the same time an outsider and an insider. An outsider in the sense that he originated outside the group, and has not entirely lost his ability to become an outsider again. An insider in the sense that his position inside the group is dependent on his ability to import an urgently needed, and otherwise unobtainable, quality into the group.

The outside-insidedness of the trader's relationship to the group and to its members produces a specific form of interaction. Wolff translates Simmel (1950: 402–406) as saying:

> He is not radically committed to the unique ingredients and peculiar tendencies of the group, and therefore approaches them with the specific attitude of objectivity. . . .

> He often receives the most surprising openness—confidences which sometimes have the character of the confessional and which would be carefully withheld from a more closely related person. . . .

> The proportion of nearness and remoteness which gives him the character of objectivity, also finds practical expression in the more abstract nature of the relation to him.

As one can see, Simmel's analysis of the trader's relationship to his client group is strikingly similar to the relationship between any professional helper and his or her client-population.

The nurse's position in relationship to her patient-population is similar to the outside-insidedness of the trader's position in relationship to his client group. The nurse is an outsider in the sense that she is not a patient. She becomes an insider inasmuch as she imports an urgently needed quality, nursing action. Nursing action does not and cannot stem from the patient-population itself. The nurse, as far as her patient-population is concerned, is an outside-insider. Her outside-insidedness produces a specific form of interaction so similar to that of the trader that by changing "he" to "she" and "his" to "her," and by substituting "patient-population" for "group," Simmel's comments exactly fit the nurse.

> (She) often receives the most surprising openness—confidences which sometimes have the character of the confessional and which would be carefully withheld from a more closely related person.

An explanation of the sudden and abruptly terminated periods of tremendous intimacy, on the part of the patient, that characterize most nurse-patient relationships.

> The proportion of nearness and remoteness which gives (her) the character of objectivity, also finds practical expression in the more abstract nature of the relationship to (her).

One wonders whether this functions to make it easier for patients to demand, to receive, and to appear to forget the "confessional phases" of the nurse-patient relationship. One also wonders whether the "abstract" nature of the patient's relationship to the nurse makes it easier for the patient to accept intimate physical care from her.

> (She) is not radically committed to the unique ingredients and peculiar tendencies of the (patient-population), and therefore approaches them with the specific attitude of objectivity.

Undoubtedly the secret of the seasoned practitioner's apparently superhuman ability to think and act objectively despite tremendous situational pressures.

Simmel describes the role of the trader and his relationships under the label "sociological stranger." Simmel's identification of the trader as a special kind of stranger helps us to understand the dynamics of the role. The trader's objectivity, which stems from his origin outside the group, is most readily understandable in terms of our own experienced objectivity on confronting an unfamiliar situation as newcomer or outsider. The confessional phenomenon is another experience that most of us have garnered in those transitional situations in which strangers meet and speak to each other. How many of us have neither confessed ourselves nor been confessed to in the safe anonymity of a bus station, an airport, or a train? And, as we remember our own experiences as strangers, we begin to understand exactly what Simmel means when he talks about the trader's role uniquely combining an extremely remote social distance with an extremely close social distance. Our own experiences as strangers also help us to realize that these two unique social distances could not be sustained in permanent, private relationships.

Although our own experiences as strangers and newcomers help us to understand Simmel's analysis of the trader, the introduction of the word *stranger* makes us uneasy about using the trader as an analytic model for any health specialist, including the nurse. The word *stranger* awakens archaic memories of the stranger as unpredictable and, therefore, dangerous. It is only natural that the use of the word should make us uneasy. If the trader is a potentially dangerous stranger, he must be abandoned;

if, on the other hand, the trader is trustworthy, our present profitable relationship with him may continue.

In order to discover whether or not the trader is trustworthy, we must examine the dynamics of a closed-group's ability to tolerate an outsider as an integral part of its social system. Closed groups characteristically reject outsiders, and it is clear from Simmel's description of the trader that both the group and the trader contributed a quality to the situation that made it possible for the trader to become an outside-insider. The group ceased to be self-sufficient by recognizing a need it could not meet with its own resources: the position in which patients characteristically find themselves. The trader demonstrated his ability to import some quality into the situation that enabled the group to meet its new need: the situation in which the nurse characteristically finds herself.

When the relationship between the trader and his client group is reduced to its initial phase, it becomes quite obvious that a combination of testing for and demonstrating mutual trustworthiness is the only possible circumstance under which a trader-closed group alliance could persist long enough to become the type of relationship Simmel describes. One could even argue that the level of trustworthiness demanded from the trader, as outside-insider, would be at a higher level than that expected from birthright members. Birthright members belong to the group, and they are never forced to leave except for the gravest misdemeanor or the grossest violation of trustworthiness. The trader, on the other hand, came from outside the group, and he would be forced out again unless he continued to demonstrate an adequate level of trustworthiness. It seems safe to say that the trader must appear to the client group to be an exceptionally trustworthy person if he is allowed to enter and become an integral part of the group's social system.

It seems to me that our need to demonstrate that the sociological stranger is trustworthy makes the trader model more suitable for our purposes. It helps us to recognize that the nurse-patient relationship also is based on the nurse's demonstration of trustworthiness. The patient's relationship with the physician is based on the patient's surrender of his pathology to the physician. The patient will not surrender his pathology unless he believes that he is surrendering it to a competent and trustworthy person. The patient does not surrender his pathology to the nurse. The patient's relationship with the nurse is based on his recognition that the nurse can, and will, provide the nursing action that he needs. If the patient is unable to trust the nurse in these matters, a nurse-patient relationship does not, and cannot, develop.

Simmel's trader as an analytic model for the relationship between the nurse and her patient-population is useful for a number of reasons. It fits extremely neatly, and with each closer examination, it demonstrates a new dimension of usefulness. It helps us to draw a sharp distinction between the nurse's private or personal relationships and the nurse's public or therapeutic relationships. It helps us to understand the patient's abrupt changes from extreme nearness, the confessional phenomenon, to extreme remoteness. It gives us a new understanding of a common, patient practice, testing for trustworthiness. It helps us to see that the nurse's actions have two functions. Not only are they therapeutic measures but also they demonstrate the nurse's trustworthiness or lack of it. It seems to me that as a model for the relationship between the nurse and her patient-population, Simmel's trader is extremely productive. All the points made so far in our argument would hold true in hospitals, clinics, and public health departments. Would it be equally useful to highly particularized nurse-patient relationships? In all probability, the most stringent test of the trader model would be to see how it stands up to the task of increasing our understanding of the relationship between the nurse and a pediatric patient.

At first glance, one is inclined to reject the trader model. The pediatric patient is a youngster separated from his family. The infant's natural environment is the mother; the young child's natural environment is the family, and the older child is still dependent, to a greater or lesser extent, on the family. Under these circumstances, one tends to assume that the constellation of relationships offered to patients by the pediatric staff should be modeled on the family in order to enable the patients to get what they need from these relationships. It is true that the pediatric staff must provide certain *services* for its patients that are usually provided by the family. The question is: Will these services be provided most effectively when the pediatric staff follow a family relationship model, or will it be more productive for them to follow the trader model?

As we have seen, invoking the trader's role helps the nurse to remain objective, and to invite the confessional phenomenon. It helps her to understand and tolerate the patient's abrupt change from intimacy to extreme remoteness. It alerts her to see that her relationships with her patients are built as she demonstrates that she can be trusted to import urgently needed nursing action into the relationship. It also has been suggested that when the nurse permits the patient to relate to her, as if she were a stranger, the patient's ability to accept necessary care and dependency is increased. Will the trader provide equally useful insights about the nurse's relationship with pediatric patients?

The pediatric patient, except in rare instances, is not seeking substitute family relationships. The pediatric patient needs substitute family services, and minimized separation from family relationships. It seems to me that the trader model helps to clarify the pediatric nurse's role in two significant ways. It permits her to remain adequately objective in a situation in which it is extremely difficult to be objective. In addition, it prevents her from displacing the mother in a situation in which she frequently must act as a mother would act.

Adults are characteristically protective toward children. All adults feel some responsibility for all children, particularly a very young child. It is difficult for most adults not to interfere when a mother seems to be mishandling or abusing her child. This characteristic response has tremendous survival value for the species, but it does create a two-edged sword for the pediatric nurse. On the one hand, it makes it possible, and in some cases rewarding, to work with critically sick and extremely unattractive children. On the other hand, it makes it difficult for her to remain detached enough to function in her public capacity as a nurse.

The relationship between the pediatric nurse and her patient has a built-in pitfall. The nurse is an adult with strong and natural feelings of protectiveness toward the young. She is an adult who may not have displaced, sublimated, or satisfactorily internalized the frustrations encountered during her own childhood. Pediatric patients come from a number of different family cultures only some of which practice the child-rearing style that the nurse has been conditioned and taught to recognize as "good." Current child-rearing attitudes place the responsibility for successful child-rearing on the child's parents, and they do not recognize that most parents are experts about their own children's idiosyncrasies. Consequently, all hospital specialists who deal with the pediatric patient tend to assume that the parents are somehow at fault because their child is sick. This unconscious attitude makes it particularly difficult for the pediatric nurse to sustain her public role as nurse. She does things for her patients that a mother does for her child, and she sometimes forgets that she is not the patient's mother.

Is it dangerous for the pediatric nurse to forget that she is not the patient's mother? On many occasions the pediatric nurse acts as the mother of the patient would act if she were present and permitted to act. On all these occasions, it is tremendously important for the nurse to remember that she is acting in her public capacity as a nurse. It is important for the nurse because it helps her to avoid replacing the mother, displacing her own childhood frustrations on the mother, and blaming the mother for the child's condition. Avoiding obvious traps in her relationship with the patient's mother enables the pediatric nurse to remain sufficiently objective to function as a nurse rather than as a foster mother. It also helps her to decrease the patient's sense of separation from family by actively including the family, whether its members are present or absent, in those transactions that are usually the function of family relationships. The nurse's ability to act as the mother would act without becoming the mother or belittling the mother is important to the pediatric patient. It is important because it does not increase his sense of separation from family by confusing him with subtle and extraneous suggestions about his relationship with his own mother.

Simmel's trader could be used with equal effect as a model for all therapist-patient relationships. The unique combination of social distances that characterize the trader's relationship with his closed group of clients are functional in any therapist-client relationship. That the relationship is based on the therapist's ability to provide a service that the patient cannot produce for himself also is true of all therapeutic relationships. All therapists build their relationships with their patients by demonstrating trustworthiness as well as competence. And the competent therapist who seems to his patient untrustworthy in therapeutic matters destroys the therapeutic character of the relationship.

The trader can be put to an additional use. It can help us to understand all relationships that must become instantly functional. In the public world of business and professional relationships, we cannot afford to impede the institution's ability to function by taking extended periods of time to accept a new colleague. And we cannot afford to mourn inordinately for the dearly departed incumbent of an adjacent office. Our failure to differentiate the social distances that characterize public-sector relationships trom those that characterize private-sector relationships, sometimes make us feel less than honest both with our colleagues and our clients.

In the public sector of our lives, we need to identify and feel comfortable with the unique combination of social distances that permit us to function effectively in institutions which are organized to permit the rapid substitution of one individual for another. We also need to assure ourselves that we are genuine in these instantly mobilized and abruptly terminated relationships. Simmel's (1950) analysis of the "sociological stranger" has helped us to identify and to understand a combination of social distances that seem productive in the public sector of our lives. Jourard[3] suggests a way in which we can determine whether or not we are acting like real people in our public-sector relationships.

[3] S. M. Jourard, *The Transparent Self* (Princeton, N.J.: D. Van Nostrand Company, Inc., 1964).

12

Self-Disclosure
and Self-Concealment

In *The Transparent Self,* Jourard [1] issues an invitation to authenticity. He invites us to come out from behind our masks and reveal ourselves to each other. He shows us how our relationships with family and with friends are diminished when we conceal ourselves from others. He suggests that the therapeutic relationship is more effective when the therapist responds as a real person, and seeks out the real person in his patient. Jouraurd talks about the bedside manner that some nurses put on when they get into their uniforms, and he shows that the nurse who approaches the patient from behind a mask tends to remain unaware of crucial problems that the patient is confronting.

The nurse who puts on a bedside manner does so in order to prevent herself from becoming too involved with the patient as a person. The bedside manner is a protective response. The nurse who hides behind the bedside manner does not understand how to build public-sector relation-

[1] S. M. Jourard, *The Transparent Self* (Princeton, N.J.: D. Van Nostrand Company, Inc., 1964).

ships, and she substitutes a mask for a relationship. All of us grew up with a net of private-sector relationships, and we frequently attempt to develop the same type of relationships with the partners assigned to us in the institutions in which we work although we know that enforced work relationships and voluntary social relationships are somewhat different.

Our private-sector relationships with family and friends are built to last. They are assumed to be permanent, and they persist through absences and for a considerable period after the death of one partner. Private-sector relationships tend to develop slowly even when the two partners are strongly attracted to each other. Public-sector relationships could be called instant relationships. They are established to serve a specific purpose. In many cases, partners are arbitrarily assigned to each other, and it is expected that the relationship will begin to be productive immediately. Public-sector relationships terminate abruptly; in some cases, one partner is replaced by another partner, and in other cases the purpose for which the relationship was established has been served, and that particular relationship is no longer needed. Because of these differences, the social distances of public- and private-sector relationships are different. It is possible to have both a private- and a public-sector relationship with the same person. And, as we shall see, it is possible to be authentic in public-sector relationships.

In both sectors there are peer relationships, and relationships in which one individual is subordinate to another. In both sectors self-disclosure and self-concealment play somewhat different roles in these two differently balanced relationships. Peer relationships develop by a balanced exchange of information about self. A relationship in which one partner has either superior position or authority uses a different balancing system, and we will examine these two balancing systems by comparing the development of a friendship with the development of a therapist-patient relationship.

A friendship is built slowly. The temptation to plunge into the relationship is resisted by both partners, and a balanced exchange of information about the real self is maintained. Each partner peels off layers of self-concealment until the most reticent partner's area of essential privacy has been delineated. The depth or openness of the relationship is determined by the most reticent partner. When the self-disclosure status quo has been established, what we might call routine self-disclosure begins. The partners routinely keep each other up to date about changes that occur in each previously disclosed category of intimate information about self.

Before the self-disclosure status quo has been established, potential imbalances exist. If a balanced exchange of intimate information is not maintained, the partner who has provided the least intimate information has potential power over the partner who has provided the most intimate information. One partner is now in the position to damage the other partner without courting an equivalent reprisal. This potential power may never be used, but the possibility that it could be used tends to change the relationship. Another possible imbalance becomes a reality when either, one or both partners, discloses items of information that they may later regret having disclosed. Imbalances also are created when one partner inadvertently discloses intimate information about the other to a third person.

After the self-disclosure, status quo has been established, internal and external pressures have the potential to create imbalances. In some cases, these pressures test the relationship, and make both partners feel more secure within the status quo that was originally established. In other cases, the status quo changes. Withdrawal, gradual or abrupt, may occur. The relationship may terminate; it may stabilize at a less intimate level, or the withdrawal may be temporary. The change may be in the other direction; both partners may open new self-discipline categories by peeling off new layers of self-concealment. In this case, either one partner's or both partners' area of essential privacy would have decreased as far as this particular relationship is concerned. Each change in self-disclosure pattern changes the individual's area of essential privacy.

Self-disclosure patterns differ from individual to individual, and they are different in the same individual during different periods of the life cycle and in different situations. A child's self-disclosure pattern is quiet different from an adult's self-disclosure pattern. An individual's self-disclosure pattern may change even in adulthood when such patterns are usually well established. An individual's self-disclosure pattern is different with different people, in different kinds of relationships and in different situations. Each change in these patterns changes the individual's areas of essential privacy. These changes sometimes make us uncomfortable with those whom we have known intimately during previous periods of our lives. An excellent example of this phenomenon is a woman's discomfort when she encounters a man with whom she played "doctors and nurses" when they were both children. "Doctors and Nurses" is a childhood game that gives children an opportunity to explore each other's bodies. By adulthood in our society some parts of the body have become areas of essential privacy as far as most relationships are concerned.

Self-disclosure and self-concealment play a somewhat different role in unequal partnerships like the therapist-patient relationship. The therapist has authority and some measure of power over the patient. In this relationship, one partner has a need that the other partner is sanctioned to meet. A functional relationship has been established to permit this process to occur. When this relationship is a temporary, public-sector relationship, it must become productive rapidly. And in most cases, it is terminated abruptly. In these functional relationships the partner with the need, patient or child, may not be able to conceal areas of privacy that are essential to him because it may be necessary for the need-meeting partner to intrude into this area in order to acomplish the primary purpose of the relationship. It may be necessary for the therapist to invade the patient's physical, psychic, and social privacy. In functional relationships of this type, the partner with the need is vulnerable, and he may not be able to conceal himself as adequately as he would wish.

The patient-therapist relationship is not developed by a balanced exchange of information. It is initiated either when a beginning is arbitrarily arranged by the institution, or when the sick person decides to seek medical help. In the latter case, the patient selects an initial partner, otherwise neither partner has much choice as far as selecting partners is concerned. A friendship is established by a balanced exchange of information about self, and it is maintained by keeping established self-disclosure categories current. A therapist-patient relationship uses a different set of balancers. In such a relationship, there are three primary balancers. The extent to which the receiving partner's needs are met; the extent to which the individual patient's sense of privacy is invaded, and the extent to which the need-meeting partner responds to the receiving partner in a straightforward and honest manner.

In a therapist-patient relationship, the therapist has the authority to dictate terms, and the patient may feel that these dicates are impositions. This sense of imposition may not be due to the terms dictated by the therapist. The receiving partner may have been forced into the role. Patients rarely seek sickness. That one partner has authority over the other partner, and that the weaker partner may have been put into the relationship against his will combine to place the burden of developing a productive relationship on the therapist.

The style of individual therapist-patient relationships is determined by the idiosyncrasies of both partners. What are the needs of the receiving partner? To what extent can this partner profit from the need-meeting partner's ability to meet needs? What is the patient's sense of essential privacy? Does the therapist usually circumvent privacy, or is it usual practice for the therapist to confront it? How sensitive are both partners in this matter of privacy? The answers to these questions characterize the style of individual therapist-patient relationships.

Privacy does not have universal boundaries. It is violated only when it appears to the individual concerned to have been violated. Particular areas of privacy seem to be essential to particular individuals, and this idiosyncratic sense of privacy must seem to be violated before damage can be done. When privacy is circumvented rather than confronted, there is less danger of damage. When privacy seems to be unnecessarily invaded, the damage done exceeds the extent of the infringement. When the patient feels that his position at the receiving end of the relationship has been arbitrarily imposed, his sense of invasion of privacy increases. When the therapist seems unaware that privacy has been invaded, the patient's sense of violation increases. Areas of essential privacy vary enormously from subculture to subculture, from individual to individual, and from one situation to another in the same individual. These variations make it difficult for the therapist to maintain the balances that make therapist-patient relationships productive.

The therapist-patient relationship is a public-sector relationship, and it has been my observation that it seems most productive when it is characterized by the social distances described in the last chapter. The unique combination of social distances that characterize the trader-closed group relationship seem to permit the therapist to remain objective without ceasing to act like a real person. They also invite the confessional phenomenon, which decreases the danger of violating the patient's sense of privacy. An understanding of these distances helps the therapist to realize that the patient's abrupt shifts from intimacy to distance are neither rejections by the patient nor failures on the part of the therapist. My observations suggest that Jourard (1964) is right. When the therapist responds as a real person, and seeks out the real person in the patient, the therapeutic relationship becomes more productive. An understanding of the dynamics of the relationship and of the social distances that characterize it makes it unnecessary for the therapist to hide behind a mask.

When the therapist leaves the institution that organizes the sick person into an instant therapist-patient relationship, and attempts to develop health-promoting programs in the community, a somewhat different set of dynamics comes into play. Members of the potential-client group take the initiative by approaching, by volunteering information about themselves, and by seeking help. The relationship is not instantly contrived in an institution; it is built up gradually by an exchange of intimate information about the client's need for advice and help from the therapist. In many ways the dynamics of the therapist-client relationship are similar to those seen in a developing friendship. That these therapist-client relationships tend to develop to the point at which the client begins to mobilize community resources to help solve the therapist's professional problems [2] suggests that an exchange of mutual assistance tends to keep these relationships in balance. The client group and their families are merely potential patients, and the client group establishes a voluntary association with the therapist.

In a hospital and in other institutional settings, an understanding of the social dynamics of the relationships, situations, and systems one encounters

[2] An example of this phenomenon is described in detail later in this book.

places the therapist in a superior position to function effectively. That hospital specialists are able to function without such understanding is obvious. It has been my observation that all those who work in hospitals do not have a working knowledge of the hospital as a dynamic social system. When therapists move into the community to promote health, they no longer are supported by a system designed for the sole purpose of enabling them to produce diagnosis, treatment, and care. Under these circumstances an understanding of social dynamics becomes a functional necessity, and I will devote the rest of *In Horizontal Orbit* to suggesting how this understanding might be developed and used.

Part Three

SOCIETY AND THE HOSPITAL: THE ROLES AND RELATIONSHIPS THEY PRODUCE

13

Society

The hospital culture described thus far was produced during attempts to implement knowledge about the unhealthy human. Space program spin-off has provided us with a considerable body of knowledge about the healthy human. If this knowledge is to be implemented, the gap between the hospital and the community must be bridged in order to enable professional health workers to function as effectively in the community as they currently function in hospitals. I intend to devote the remaining chapters of *In Horizontal Orbit* to a brief sketch of our society and to speculations about how a bridge might be constructed.

American society could be classified as western industrial, but it differs from most western industrial societies in the way in which it has recruited its membership. Most societies depend for new membership almost entirely on the birthrate, whereas our society is a European transplant into which large numbers of persons from many countries have been assimilated. One of the most interesting things about it is the way in which a population with diverse ethnic backgrounds has produced a society with unique characteristics and a culture of its own. The United States is called a melting-pot society; this label has reference to the overt and vigorous way in which we Americanize immigrants. That one of the techniques used has been sucessful is testified to by two extracts from my field diary: the first recorded in Germany in 1945; and the second in this country in 1960.

German Extract, 1945

Three of the four American members of the team (UNRRA) grew up with parents who were more comfortable speaking other languages (Russian, Polish, Czechoslovakian). All three of them speak flawless English, and need interpreters when they work with displaced persons who speak the language native to their own parents. It seems a pity that these bilingual opportunities were avoided rather than capitalized.

American Extract, 1960

Dr. Y pays Mr. F to translate letters to and from his mother. She is old and has forgotten the English words she used while rearing him, and he has forgotten most of the Polish words he heard while he was being reared.

These two observations comment on one of the many ways in which new members of the society are encouraged to abandon characteristics that might differentiate them from birthright members of the society.

The dominant segment of American society has industrialized rapidly and, as far as the rise in material level is concerned, extremely successfully. It is an urban society characterized by geographically and economically mobile nuclear families; large-scale organizations designed to either produce goods and services or to process people; and residency patterns that suggest this segment of the society is separating itself into a socioeconomic hierarchy characterized by visible consumption patterns rather than ethnic differences. I call this segment of American society the "launching-pad" society because its family structure is designed to produce, to rear, and to launch one set of offspring. When I diagram the launching-pad society, it looks like the drawing in Figure 6.

In this diagram the large-scale institutions are separated into two categories: those that produce goods and services and those that process people. I call the institutions that do things to people, people-processing plants; and I identify three kinds of people-processing plants: launching plants—schools, colleges, and other institutions that prepare people to become working members of society; fall-out plants—institutions that do something to and for people when they are *temporarily* unable to function in society (hospitals and prisons fall into this category); and scrap institutions—the institutions in which we store human rejects (homes for the retarded and nursing homes for the aged are both excellent examples).

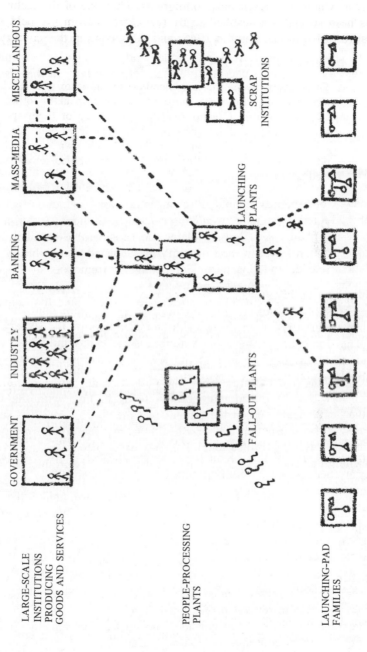

Figure 6. The launching-pad society. (An elaboration of a diagram presented in a lecture by Solon T. Kimball [1962]).

It is curious that we frequently use the word "home" in the names we attach to our scrap institutions.

The small squares in the bottom row of Figure 6 represent what I call the launching-pad family.[1] The launching-pad family is an adaptation to rapid change. It is extremely mobile, and it courts rather than resists change. The launching-pad family is characterized later in this chapter, and the way in which it responds to and uses professional health workers is discussed at some length.

The large-scale institutions that produce goods and services have produced an unprecedented rise in material level in Western societies since the beginning of the Industrial Revolution. These institutions and our people-processing-plants model themselves on the mass-production factory, the most visibly successful goods-producing institution in an industrial society. Consequently, significant changes in mass-production factories tend to be adopted eventually by *all* large-scale institutions, including people-processing plants. As I have explained in considerable detail in an earlier chapter, the mass-production factory has started a revolution in organizational style, and this particular change is tremendously important to all people-processing plants, including the hospital.

Although all segments of our society do not look like the launching-pad society, the dominant segment of American society is organized in this manner, and this segment tends to assimilate the more mobile members from other segments. The frame of reference within which the physician, the nurse, and other professional health workers function is a product of the launching-pad culture. When the patient is an active member of the subsociety that produced that culture, he is in tune with the intentions of the health team. When the patient is a member of an alien subculture, he may either misunderstand the health team's intentions or resist them. In either case the professional health worker needs to understand our launching-pad society, and the unique subculture it is producing. This need becomes clear when we think about the health-related implications of ethnic differences and of family structures that are unlike the structure of families in the dominant segment of our society. We will look first at family structure.

In all societies the family is the basic social system. Although it can be, and is, organized in a number of different ways not only in different societies but also in different subcultures within our own society, most of us think of the family in which we ourselves were reared as what a family should be. Health-related professionals tend to come from the dominant segment of the society and consider the nuclear or launching-pad family "normal." As a consequence extended families and matrifocal families

---

[1] I discovered after I coined this phrase that Margaret Mead speaks of the separated nuclear family as a "launching-platform." I am delighted that my own mind tends to leap in such excellent company.

sometimes create problems that physicians, nurses, and other professional health workers must solve.

An extended family system is found in the Cracker culture, described in the next chapter, and it has been my observation that this family system creates a hospital visiting problem and interferes with scientific child-rearing. Hospital visiting rules have been designed to accommodate the visiting patterns of the nuclear family, and the large-group visiting of the sick which characterizes the Cracker extended family is difficult for many nurses and physicians to tolerate. In this family system, it is customary for older and experienced women to assist with and offer advice about child-rearing. Child-rearing specialists consider much of this advice outmoded, and when it is readily available, as it is in a viable extended family system, it sometimes prevents the biological mother from carrying out the pediatrician's child-rearing instructions. Hospital regulations and the problem-solving approaches of hospital specialists tend to be designed on the assumption that all families are nuclear, launching-pad families. A matrifocal family system is found at lower socioeconomic levels in our society. As we shall see, it may be a productive adaptation to a particular ecological niche in spite of most professional helpers thinking of it as a broken family with an unstable head, an evaluation that suggests problems that may not exist. I will begin my discussion of these three different family systems by comparing the launching-pad family and the matrifocal family. The launching-pad family has detached itself from a bilateral extended family, and it will be described during our examination of the launching-pad family.

The structure of family systems can be diagramed by using circles to represent females, and triangles to represent males. Space and lines are used to describe relationships between family members. If each family included one son and one daughter, the two family systems would appear as shown in Figure 7.

From Figure 7, we can see that the launching-pad family and the matrifocal family are organized in a somewhat different manner. As we shall see, *both* family systems are productive adaptations to different sets of conditions. These two facts have practical implications for all categories of health specialists. Patients do not exist in a social vacuum. For the most part they are members of families, and in many cases their health problems cannot be understood and dealt with unless this is taken into consideration. Those in the health professions tend to come from segments of American society in which families are organized in a manner similar to the way in which the launching-pad family is organized. As a consequence, they sometimes fail to recognize the matrifocal family as a productive adaptation to a particular set of conditions. This failure can, and sometimes does, prevent the solution of health problems.

Just as I began my study of the hospital by identifying its central func-

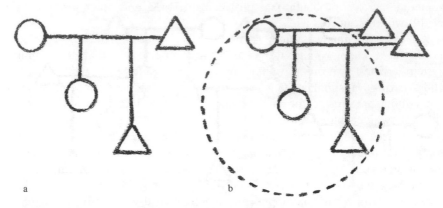

Figure 7. (a) The launching-pad family; (b) matrifocal family.

tion so we must begin our examination of these two family systems by identifying the central function of the family. As we are comparing two different family systems, we will need to use a function that holds true for all families in all societies. The social functions performed by the family vary from society to society, but in all societies the family functions to place the children it produces in a recognized position in the social system.[2] We will use this function when we characterize and compare the launching-pad family and the matrifocal family.

The launching-pad family has emerged from the dominant kinship system in our society. The dominant kinship system in America is organized around a nuclear unit that consists of a set of parents and their children. This nuclear unit is organized around a husband-wife axis, and the kinship system to which it belongs includes both parents' blood lines; it is a bilateral kinship system. Those who belong to this kinship system say: "I am an X on my father's side of the family, and a Y on my mother's side of the family" (see Figure 8).

The launching-pad family is a nuclear unit that separates itself from such a kinship system. What the dominant segment of American society has defined as "marriage" gives the children of the launching-pad family and the extended family a recognized position in society.

The launching-pad family is an adaptation to the need for rapid change. It establishes social, and frequently geographical, distance between itself and both families of origin. It practices scientifically determined child-rearing, and it characteristically avoids those who might encourage it to use old fashioned or traditional child-rearing practices. It tends to live in a series of single-class neighborhoods rather than in the mixed neighbor-

[2] B. Malinowski, "Parenthood—the basis of social structure" in *The New Generation*. V. F. Calverton and Schmalhsusen, eds. (New York: Macaulay Company, 1930). See chapter notes for extended discussion.

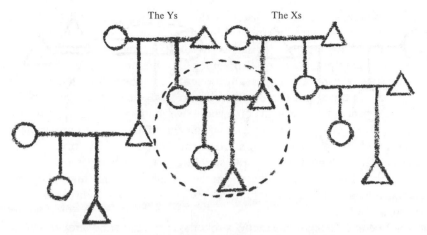

Figure 8. Extended family, American model.

hoods in which the extended family tended to live. It is geographically and socially mobile; it moves readily from place to place and from socioeconomic level to socioeconomic level; and it tends to sever social relationships as it moves either up or down in the socioeconomic hierarchy. When it moves, it may strip itself down to bare essentials: its car or cars, best clothes, prized possessions, bank balance, and credit rating, leaving behind discarded furniture and abandoned relationships. The launching-pad family is like a chameleon in that it rapidly becomes indistinguishable in new social surroundings. It is obvious that many nuclear families in our society have not separated sufficiently from the extended family to qualify as launching-pad families, but this type of family is emerging as a preferred model in the dominant segment of our society. The maternal and child-care practices advocated by health specialists have been designed to conform to these values and to meet the needs of this family system.

The classical example of a separated nuclear family most similar to our own launching-pad family is the polar Eskimo family. The polar Eskimos are said to group into small clusters of nuclear families.[3] Their clustering patterns are organized on a voluntary association basis rather than according to kinship. These clusters of families vary in size, depending on the resources available during different seasons of the year. Two or three during the summer when the caribou is hunted, seven or eight during the winter, and in somewhat larger clusters during the spring. Their habit of clustering in groups of separated nuclear families on a voluntary association basis is similar to the grouping behavior of the launching-pad family. The primary difference is that our affluent environment permits considerably larger clusters.

The environment in which the polar Eskimo lives does not allow more

[3] K. Birket-Smith, *The Eskimos* (New York: E. P. Dutton & Co., Inc., 1936).

than a few dozen people to cluster in the same place; in addition, it does not permit one person to maintain himself as a single unit. Consequently, unattached adults attach themselves to existing nuclear families. Their people-scrapping practices are also somewhat different from our own. The Eskimo society cannot support unproductive members for any considerable period of time, and those who fall into this category are jettisoned in order to ensure the survival of productive and potentially productive members. It is interesting that an environment which cannot support large groupings of people and an environment which comfortably supports extremely large groupings of people should produce societies with so much in common. Both societies have similar family systems and clustering patterns that are based on voluntary association rather than on kinship. The social solution for bachelors and spinsters may be quite different, but the people-scrapping practices of the two societies are somewhat similar.

For the most part, physicians, nurses, social workers, teachers and other professional helpers were reared in family systems similar to the polar Eskimo nuclear family and the launching-pad family. Consequently, they tend to assume that this type of family is the only "normal" family. This assumption and many of the practices of those who work with families in our society are based on the notion that *all* families should be organized in this manner. As we shall see, all "normal" families in our society are not separated nuclear families organized around a husband-wife axis. Failure to recognize this, sometimes interferes with the professional helper's ability to function effectively. These failures tend to become visible as attempts to interfere with extended family supports and influences and as decisions based on the assumption that the matrifocal family is a broken family.[4]

The launching-pad family is an adaptation to rapid change in affluent segments of our society and the matrifocal family is an adaptation to sparse economic opportunities in some of the least affluent parts of our society. In the matrifocal family, the mather and her children are organized into a stable unit, and the biological father is an in-and-out person who does not have a permanent position in the family he fathers although he does have a permanent position in his family of origin and in the community. Among peoples that organize their families in this manner, biological fathers contribute to the support of their children, and adult males contribute to the support of their mothers. Males establish strong relationships with their same-sex-age peers and with workmates. Contrary to common assumption, there is no lack of male-role models for young male members in these segments of our society.

[4] For a discussion of the broken family, *see* E. L. Koos, *Families in Trouble* (New York: Kings Crown Press, 1946).

The matrifocal family is not unique to the least affluent segments of industrial societies. It is found, for example, in the Caribbean [5] where major portions of the population are organized in this manner. When we compare the socioeconomic situation in which our own matrifocal families are found with the socioeconomic situation of those segments of Caribbean society in which matrifocal families are found, we begin to realize that this particular family system is an excellent adaptation to an ecological niche in which multiple subsistence opportunities must be exploited in order to ensure survival. The matrifocal family seems to appear in situations in which a number of different economic opportunities must be exploited, and in situations in which it is advantageous for the male to remain relatively mobile if the community is to survive. From the point of view of those in more affluent segments of our own society, matrifocal families seem to be either pathological or immoral. A great deal of well-intentioned nonsense characterizes the way in which those, who work with and try to help these families, think and talk about matrifocal families.

The matrifocal family is the most frequently misinterpreted family in our society, partly because it is difficult to get accurate information about the various ways in which the subsociety that produces the matrifocal family organizes itself to confront the world in which it lives, and partly because we use an alien yardstick to measure it. I am suggesting that the matrifocal family is neither pathological nor immoral. It is merely a system of family organization that is characteristically found when a particular set of subsistence opportunities is present. My observations suggest that the matrifocal family at lower socioeconomic levels in American society may be a productive adaptation to the need to exploit multiple subsistence opportunities.

The so-called illegitimacy rate in these segments of the society is an excellent example of an alien yardstick distortion. In all societies, the function of the family is to make children legitimate members of the society (Malinkowski 1930). In the subsociety that produces our own matrifocal family, periods of common residence by the biological parents ensures that the child of this union will be recognized as a legitimate member of the subsociety, even though this form of "marriage" is not recognized as legitimate by the dominant segment of the society. As far as our own matrifocal families are concerned, their need to exploit the welfare system contributes to our confusion about illegitimacy rates and increases the apparent desertion rate.[6] It is interesting that in some states,

[5] W. J. Goode, "Illegitimacy in the Caribbean Social Structures," *Amer. Sociol. Rev.* 25 (1960): 21–30.

[6] Changes suggested by President Nixon, August 1969, should decrease the apparent desertion rate.

we recognize the legality of common-residence unions and common-law marriage when property is at stake.

Let me describe the matrifocal family as I have seen it in a number of contemporary Western societies. It is an adaptation to multiple subsistence opportunities; it tends to be geographically stable; it consists of a mother and her children; it survives at subsistence level; it is cohesive, and all members contribute to its support as soon as possible. The maternal grandmother, and in some cases great-grandmother, tends to rear the children, primarily because the economic opportunities of a younger woman are superior to those of an older woman. In these segments of our society, women are considered productive members until they are almost totally incapacitated. When one examines the populations in nursing homes, one discovers that the number of men from lower socioeconomic backgrounds is three or four times as great as the number of women from similar backgrounds. Those at higher socioeconomic levels seem to scrap men and women at an equal rate, but because women tend to live longer, slightly more women than men are inmates of the nursing homes patronized by the more affluent segments of American society.[7]

The matrifocal family is embedded in a community in which adult males are firmly based although they may leave the community periodically to seek temporary employment. The male child does not lack male role models. And peer relationships begin early, and continue to be important during the entire life span, particularly for male members. This subsociety uses the sidewalk and other common meeting places in much the same way as launching-pad families use their homes and their clubs. Whyte describes this subsociety in his book *The Street Corner Society*.[8] The notion that people in street-corner societies lack "home life" misinterprets their social behavior. In our society families at lower socioeconomic levels use houses to sleep in, to eat in, and to keep things in. In many ways street-corner living provides a richer environment than the hothouse homes of our launching-pad families.

American middle-class bias about the matrifocal family might be adjusted more readily if we were to consider other ecological niches in our society that have produced outcroppings of females who tend to organize their families in a matrifocal fashion. Sailing ships and the economy of seafaring created a social situation that tended to produce females culturally conditioned to function in a matrifocal manner; and although wooden ships have disappeared, the cultural tradition persists. Certain occupations, show business, for example, produce subcultures in which

[7] Information collected while acting as consultant to the Public Health Department, State of Florida, 1960–1961.

[8] W. F. Whyte, *The Street Corner Society* (Chicago: Chicago University Press, 1943).

the matrifocal family is adaptive. In such subcultures, the matrifocal family emerges, in some cases for ethnic reasons, and in other cases as an adaptation.

Professional helpers in our society are at a disadvantage when they work with and attempt to help the members of a street-corner society. Their attempts to help are impeded by cultural barriers, and because they represent the hostile status quo. The professional helper also is at some disadvantage when working with those from any other segment of our society that has not been assimilated into the cultural mainstream. The attempt to create a unique American culture has produced many subcultures that seem alien to physicians, nurses, and other categories of professional helpers. In a very real sense, cultural barriers interfere with many of these attempts to increase the well-being of individual members of their society.

The launching-pad society is arranged in a hierarchy of socioeconomic subcultures, and it can be thought of as the mainstream of a unique American culture. It is the product of rapid technological development, and a melting-pot approach to the problem of assimilating large numbers of people from diverse ethnic backgrounds. The urban and rural populations in which our matrifocal families are found have not been absorbed into this cultural mainstream, and do not feel that they belong to the launching-pad society. In addition, at both lower and higher socioeconomic levels, there are pockets of the population that refuse to become part of this emerging culture, and who stubbornly insist on maintaining their own ethnic identities. One such subculture is described in some detail in the next chapter.

In addition to the three family systems described in this chapter, other modifications of family structure are encountered from time to time by those in the health professions. It is therefore useful to be able to identify differences in family structure. The launching-pad family is organized around a husband-wife axis, and it is detached from extended kinship networks. It becomes an impaired or broken family when the axis partnership is impaired or broken. Under similar circumstances, a nuclear unit embedded in extended family ties becomes a somewhat different proposition as far as those in the helping professions are concerned. In this case, modifications in the nuclear unit are compensated for by adjustments in the larger social system of the extended family. The matrifocal family is part of a matriarchal kinship system and it is organized around a mother-daughter axis, and tends to be found in communities where older females of necessity control many facets of community life in addition to assuming the primary responsibility for rearing the young. These facts should be taken into consideration by those who wish to improve the health of individuals who are members of this type of subculture. A fourth family system sometimes encountered is that which is organized around the father-son axis. This family is produced by a clan system in which males remain members of their clan of origin whereas females do not. We find father-son axis families in parts of our own country where a clan system imported from Scotland persists, as, for example, in some southeastern mountain areas. Patriarchies like matriarchies tend to resist change, and older members of the dominant sex control community behavior, and decide how children will be reared. In both systems sex roles are clearly defined, and the work and other behavior appropriate to each sex is differentiated.

The frame of reference of those in the health professions has been moulded by the launching-pad society, and it is sometimes difficult for physicians, nurses, and other professional health workers to communicate with and to help those from these various subcultures. When the disease is acute, medical understanding outweighs cultural misunderstanding. But as the emphasis shifts from cure to health, alien cultural barriers become increasingly difficult to surmount. In the next chapter, we will consider cultural barriers.

14

Cultural Barriers

Professional health workers tend to come from that segment of society most frequently referred to as either "middle" or "upper-middle" class, and their patients or clients come from all segments of the society. As a consequence, cultural barriers exist, and sometimes cause the help offered and the advice given to be at cross purposes. In some cases the professional helper, physician, nurse, social worker, and so forth, is thought of as a representative of the hostile status quo; and when this happens, help and advice are resented and avoided. In other cases, resistance occurs because two opposing value systems are confronting each other. In still other instances the expert's advice has not been interpreted correctly. The members of all segments of American society value the sense of well being that they recognize as health, but in some cases the cultural differences between the therapist and the client become barriers. In this chapter, we will examine our melting-pot society, and attempt to identify and characterize the cultural barriers most frequently encountered by those in the health professions.

I call our society a melting-pot society because of our approach to the problem of creating a homogenous culture out of groups of people from diverse ethnic backgrounds. This approach has produced a dominant segment of society, generally referred to as "the middle class," in which a hierarchy of socioeconomic subcultures has eradicated the surface appearance of ethnic differences. In addition to this hierarchy, there are resistant ethnic pockets and an economically disadvantaged subsociety. Some insights into this system of subcultures can be gained by an examination of changing value systems.

Veblen [1] advanced a thesis that permits us to see the changing value systems in our society as a dynamic process. Veblen contended that when traditional values are eroded by mobility and rapid rises in life standards, these values tend to be replaced by those directed toward the emulation and imitation of the economically better off. This change produces value systems based on the most visible behavior of those in superior economic positions. We should be able to trace these changes by considering the visibility of superior economic behavior. If we examine America's changing value systems from this point of view, we can identify two periods during which the opportunity to observe superior economic behavior was somewhat different: an initial period during which the visible behavior of those at superior socioeconomic levels was experienced firsthand and by hearsay and a subsequent period during which firsthand and hearsay information was supplemented and eventually dominated by mass media.

During the initial period, vigorous attempts were made to impose the bourgeois values of thrift, austerity, and production, on the working classes. These attempts failed, and an interesting theory about working-class leisure emerged as an explanation of this failure. The original hypothesis was that the form of working-class leisure was determined by the need to compensate for the deprivations of the work situation. This theory about working-class leisure seemed valid in the intellectual climate into which it was introduced, at a time when social scientists had expended considerable energy examining man's adaptation to the submachine role, and they were convinced that the submachine role was potentially lethal. Under these circumstances, it was natural that the experts should interpret the worker's refusal to "better himself" as an inability to do so, due to an overriding need to compensate for the deprivations of the work situation. Even Weber [2] who had a mathematician's delight in the elegant logic of the bureaucratic system suggests the soul-eroding impact of the bureaucratic way of life.

---

[1] T. Veblen, *The Theory of the Leisure Class: An Economic Study of Institutions* (New York: The Modern Library, 1934).

[2] From Max Weber, *Essays in Sociology,* trans. and ed. H. H. Gerth and C. W. Mills (New York: Oxford University Press, 1958, pp. 161–162).

In 1959, Pizzorno[3] offered what seems to be a more satisfactory explanation. Pizzorno suggests that working-class attempts to adopt bourgeois value systems were doomed to failure because the working-class economic situation was incompatible with a bourgeois value system. In addition, because the economic situation was incompatible, leisure values began to develop as a counter system. When we think of changing-value systems from this point of view, we begin to see that those who were attempting to impose their traditional value system on the working classes had already begun to displace this system with a leisure value system borrowed from the aristocracy.

It is now obvious that the tendency to replace eroding traditional values with leisure value systems based on the visible behavior of those in superior economic positions is not peculiar to the working classes. This tendency permeated Western societies, and our melting-pot society is, in part, a product of this tendency. Apparently Veblen (1934) was right. In all industrial societies, mobility and rapid rises in life standard tend to separate members of subcultures from their traditional value systems. At all levels in an industrial society, there seems to be a tendency to stylize life on a leisure value system based on the visible behavior of those in superior socioeconomic positions.

The introduction of the moving picture increased the visibility of the behavior of those at superior economic positions. It also homogenized the life style upon which leisure value systems were based. Television brought more of this information into the home, and virtually eradicated previous differences in media exposure. As a consequence, we now live in a society in which our value systems tend to be based on canned descriptions of how those at superior socioeconomic levels in the society supposedly spend free time and freely disposable income. In addition, the demand for consumer goods and organized amusement is manipulated in the interest of economic growth, and our everyday lives have been recreated in forms that derive from industrialism and contribute to its development.[4] The various ways in which people spend their money and time has become visible as a concrete form in which the social system is manifest in action. In other words, the subcultures in our society have become visible as characteristic consumption patterns.

Those in the health and other helping professions need to be able to identify the subcultures from which their patients and clients come. Individuals from these subcultures characteristically respond in three different ways to attempts to help them to solve their problems. It is easier to help

[3] A. Pizzorono, "Accumulation loisirs et rapports de classe." *Esprits* (June 1959).
[4] T. A. Burns, "Meaning in Everyday Life." *New Society* (May 25, 1967).

people when one understands how and why they are responding. Members of the dominant hierarchy of socioeconomic subcultures, the "middle class" American, tend to seek an actively cooperating role. Members of ethnic-pocket subcultures will cooperate within the limits determined by their own traditional value systems. Members of economically disadvantaged populations tend to regard professional helpers as agents of a hostile status quo with the authority to coerce them. These three somewhat different responses to the professional helper must be taken into consideration if the potential patient and the patient are to become active members of the health team.

The consumption patterns of the dominant hierarchy of socioeconomic subcultures in American society are characterized by conspicuous consumption and conformity, and by a tendency to permit expenditure to outstrip income in a more or less orderly manner. In this segment of our society, individual consumption patterns tend to change at each move up the socioeconomic hierarchy, and at each move from one place to another. Members of this set of subcultures value the professional helper, believe in the efficacy of his expertize, and are prepared to sacrifice time and money in order to follow professional advice. Individuals from this segment of our society are ready to become cooperating members of the health team. They fail to do so under two circumstances: when they are incapacitated, temporarily or permanently, and when they are prevented from functioning in this manner by the professional members of the health team.

Ethnic-pocket subcultures may be strikingly different from each other, but they do have a number of common characteristics. They insist on maintaining their unique ethnic identities. They resist changes that run counter to their traditional values. Their consumption patterns do not necessarily reflect leisure values borrowed from other segments of the society. However, their traditional values are being slowly eroded, and there tends to be a conflict between generations about these value changes.

Members of ethnic-pocket subcultures tend to value health professionals and the advice they give unless this advice runs counter to their beliefs. Ethnic-pocket subcultures are found at both higher and lower socioeconomic levels in our society. Their position in the economic hierarchy depends on the extent to which their solidarity and their resistance to change has enhanced their economic opportunities. Later in this chapter, I will describe an ethnic-pocket subculture that is found at both high and low socioeconomic levels in order to identify some of the problems that professional health workers encounter when they work with those from ethnic-pocket subcultures.

The subcultures of the economically disadvantaged have produced extremely interesting consumption patterns. In these segments of American society, families tend to exist at bare subsistence levels by exploiting a number of economic opportunities. In this sense, the welfare system is an economic opportunity.[5] All members of the family contribute to its support as soon as possible, and individual families experience periods of relative affluence when their children are grown and before the children establish families of their own. These brief periods of affluence are characterized by a sharp increase in the consumption of such things as food, drink, clothes, cars, television sets, organized amusement, and so forth. Although individual families exploit welfare possibilities, most members of this subculture tend to distrust professional helpers, and to avoid them if it is at all possible to do so. They also tend to fear hospitals, and this fear seems to have three sources. The hospital is a place in which they expect to die. The taxicab driver who said: "I was born in a hospital, and I expect I'll die in one," expressed a typical attitude. They believe that poor people are experimented on in hospitals, particularly teaching hospitals. This opinion was expressed by the elevator operator who advised me to avoid a hospital where "they experiment on people" and to seek another where "they let you die in peace." And they cannot entirely trust the good intentions of those who work in hospitals. When members of an economically disadvantaged subculture enter a hospital, they place themselves at the mercy of those whom they consider to be members of a hostile society. When this feeling of distrust is complicated either by race or ethnic conflicts, it can produce fear of death. Some years ago a nursing student drew my attention to the "black bottle." Patients were overheard advising other patients to behave themselves in ways that would not tempt hospital staff to use "the black bottle"; and we discovered that communities from which these patients had come believed that some of their members had been quietly disposed of by the hospital staff during the night. The lethal shot or dose was known as the "black bottle."

Full-fledged members of the launching-pad society and members of its economically disadvantaged subcultures have quite different attitudes about poverty. In the affluent segments of our society, poverty is valued as a phase through which the young adult passes on the way to success. In economically disadvantaged populations, poverty is a way of life from which it is almost impossible to escape. The first attitude is a future-oriented view of poverty, and the latter attitude is present-oriented. The

[5] In one southeastern county the various welfare agencies, including groups like the Salvation Army, were asked to rank their client families. It was interesting that the families considered "successful cases" tended to appear on more than one list. In some cases, individual families appeared on so many lists that the welfare workers who had ranked them said: "These families have made a profession out of being successful welfare cases." (This information was given to me by a public health nurse who prefers not to be mentioned by name.)

characteristic consumption patterns of the two populations reflect this difference.

In the more or less affluent segments of our society, the myth of beginning at the bottom and working one's way to the top is preserved in the poverty phase of the successful career. This particular phenomenon is collected into married student villages on college campuses, and can be readily examined by the interested observer. The consumption patterns in these villages is one of conspicuous poverty. The material resources available to the families in these villages vary enormously depending on the extent to which official income is supplemented by gifts and token loans from parents and siblings. Some families barely make ends meet by practicing the most rigid economies. At the other extreme, the "official income" is mere pocket money. In either case conspicuous poverty must seem to characterize consumption patterns. Those families which have the resources to behave in an affluent manner are at a unique disadvantage in this subculture. The housewife who is merely pretending to pinch pennies may inadvertently buy a nine-strand lawn chair rather than the seven-strander that is on the market for one dollar less. And a new car for which cash has been paid must be passed off as an acquisition for which the owner will be obligated to the loan company during the maximum number of permissible years.

When poverty is a way of life from which it is almost impossible to escape, the most conspicuous aspects of poverty are not boasted about. An informant from one of these subcultures described a scene that illustrated this difference. My informant was talking to me about a period during which she had been particularly in need: she was out of work, and she had to feed her two children and herself. One night there was nothing to eat, and she did not want her neighbors to know. She took the children into her confidence, and they boiled some water on the stove. While this feast was being prepared, my informant said: "We sang and carried on like we were cooking steak."

Those with remnants of a value system that equates godliness with affluence tend to assume that pride is absent in the poor. This misunderstanding is confirmed by a tendency to misunderstand the conspicuous consumption that characterizes periods of effluence in the life cycle of lower socioeconomic families. To those in a superior economic position, it seems unreasonable that money is thrown around as down payments on extravagances and as costly amusement when it could be invested in the future. The economically disadvantaged do not see themselves as having much of a future. They see themselves as have-nots in a society that has unprecedented material resources.

Different subcultures not only have different frames of reference but also they have different uses for expressions in the same language. Some years ago a graduate student in psychology discovered an interesting difference between upper and lower socioeconomic females. Those at lower socioeconomic levels responded to the first menstrual period physiologically while those at higher levels responded psychologically. In answer to the question "How did you feel when . . .?" those at lower socioeconomic levels described pain, the sight of blood, and so forth; whereas those at superior levels recalled their emotional reactions. When the question was reworded "What worried you about . . .?" those who had previously responded with a list of physical symptoms described their emotional reactions to the first menstrual period. For the most part the other group denied that they had been "worried," and went on to describe how they had "felt" about it.

Differences in mores sometimes cause those in the health professions to leap to middle-class conclusions. A nursing student became disturbed about a mother who had not named her new baby. She developed an elaborate theory about her patient's subconscious rejection of her sex role and her child. When the student went into the matter more deeply, she discovered that her patient was behaving in a perfectly normal manner. In the subculture to which the patient belonged, the right to name the baby belonged to a female member of the infant's maternal grandmother's generation. The child's mother customarily selected a "namer" from this group of female relatives. The "namer" selected the name of the infant and it was bestowed some weeks after birth at an elaborate ceremony in the maternal grandmother's house to which all the child's maternal kin were automatically invited. Patients from this particular subculture are forced to provide a name for the birth certificate, but it is not necessarily the name the infant actually receives, a necessity that frequently causes confusion at a later date.

In addition to this routine cultural barrier, the health worker encounters stubborn resistances that are caused by value-system conflicts. A public health nurse described this example.[6] Apparently, it is now customary to discourage the oiling of young infants, a practice that is traditional in some subcultures. The nurse was dealing with mothers who had been led to believe that oiling a baby was "good" for it. She found that it was easy to talk some of her clients out of this practice, but that others refused to follow her advice. At first she assumed that those who did not respond were stupid. Then she realized that the resisting mothers were not particularly stupid in other matters. She decided to investigate and discovered that the resisting mothers belonged to a religious group that believed olive oil had supernatural powers to protect and to heal. She talked to the "preacher" about her problem, and he suggested that she change the bathing ritual she was teaching to include an anointment with oil. From that

[6] My informant prefers not to be mentioned by name.

moment the problem ceased to exist. The mothers bathed their infants in the approved manner and instead of smothering them with oil they rubbed a drop of oil onto the forehead.

Most of the barriers that are encountered by the health professions when they work with patients from ethnic-pocket subcultures tend to be due to value system conflicts. Ethnic-pocket subcultures are actively refusing to become part of the launching-pad society. They resist changing their culture as a matter of principle, and their traditional value systems have been strengthened because they are being fought for. They value health, and in most cases they set store by scientific medicine. As patients, they are cooperative until the health specialist unwittingly triggers a value-system conflict, at which point they may become, as one physician put it: "impossible to deal with." Our ethnic-pocket subcultures are eroding rapidly, and there is a marked difference between younger and older generations. In some cases, the younger generation has already abandoned the traditional value system, and is merely appearing to conform to it. It is important for the health specialist to be able to distinguish between absolute insistence and token resistance.

There is a considerable body of literature available about most of the ethnic-pocket subcultures from which patients come. Esther Lucille Brown's [7] cultural blueprints are particularly useful to those in the health professions. To end this chapter, I am going to show how a cultural blueprint can be used by physicians, nurses, and others to increase their understanding of health problems. I will begin by blueprinting a subculture that I observed during a five-year period in the fifties, the Cracker culture. [8]

The South produced two subcultures: the plantation culture, popularized by books and movies about the South, and the Cracker culture. The Cracker culture was developed out of attempts to exploit subsistence opportunities along the waterways in the southeastern section of the country, through central South Carolina, down through Georgia, into northern and central Florida, west through Alabama, and into Louisiana. These attempts were dominated by the cultural style of Scottish and Scots-Irish immigrants, by the Calvinistic traditions, and by a frontier way of life.

In a Cracker society, relationships between individuals are based on mutual and absolute trust. A man's word is as good as his bond, and verbal agreements rather than written contracts are customary. If absolute trust breaks down, or if an individual wishes to go his own way, a complete

[7] E. L. Brown, *Newer Dimensions of Patient Care: Patients as People.* Part 3. (New York: Russell Sage Foundation, 1964). pp. 56–86.

[8] An excellent account of the "cultural mix" in which Cracker culture is embedded is found in M. Pearsall, "Cultures of the American South." *Anthro. Quart.* 39, no. 2 (1966): 128–141.

break with kin and community is made. When disagreements between family members cannot be healed, one or the other party to the disagreement either withdraws from or is dispatched out of the society.

The society is organized on an extended kinship system that is similar to a Scottish clan system. The political system is an extension of the kinship system. Originally, law and order were maintained and economic opportunities were exploited as functions of the kinship system, a pattern typical of frontier societies. Disagreements between members of two different kinship systems tend to involve all members of both clans, and to persist after those who originated the quarrel have died. A Cracker society is a closed society; outsiders are not readily accepted, and members find it difficult to tolerate strangers. There is an interesting exception to the Cracker's characteristic response to outsiders and strangers. An outsider with the same surname *may* be accepted into an extended family as a kinsman even when there is no evidence of a blood tie. When instances like this are examined, it is found that it was to the political advantage of the accepting extended family to secure additional voting power by increasing kin membership.

The Cracker is found at both lower and higher socioeconomic levels. His attitude about property and toward poverty is in contrast to the attitudes that characterize both the populations in which our launching-pad families are found, and the populations in which our urban and rural matrifocal families are found. The Cracker attitude about property and toward poverty is similar to that of the Scot. The Cracker does not indulge in conspicuous consumption. At higher socioeconomic levels, he may drive a Cadillac because it is a superior vehicle, but you will not discover by his appearance and behavior in the town square that he is a man of substance until you see him climb into his car. You will not be able to walk around town and unerringly differentiate the houses of the "rich" from the houses of the "poor." In some cases, there are differences in size, but in as much as size may be accumulated over several generations, size in itself is not a distinguishing characteristic. The condition of the outside of the house is not a reliable indicator. I have been surprised to find wall-to-wall carpeting, luxurious furnishings, and the most expensive air conditioning inside houses that looked from the outside as if their owners were in dire straits.

Among Crackers, the attitude toward official poverty, as defined by government agencies, is one of fierce independence. The Cracker expects, and gets, help from kin. This help can be repaid in the course of a generation or two, if not in the course of a single lifetime. The Cracker sets a high value on not being "beholden." He does not feel that honest poverty is anything to be ashamed of. Like the Scot, he recognizes that lack of opportunity rather than lack of ability are responsible for his economic condition. When opportunity presents itself, the Cracker takes shrewd advantage of it. The Cracker is not in tune with the "affluent society" [9] although he makes profitable use of that society's economic system when opportunities are available to him. The Cracker does not sever social relationships as he moves up in the economic hierarchy, and he does not tend to change his life style to conform to that which is considered appropriate to his economic status.

Within this subculture, the child is accepted as the natural consequence of marital relationships, and each child is assigned a specific social and economic role. The role of the boy and the role of the girl is clearly differentiated. During early childhood, children spend most of their time in their own homes or in the homes of their cousins. Fathers, grandfathers, uncles, and male cousins teach boys to be a boy and a man. The females in the extended family system teach girls how to be girls and women. Both the father and the mother are nonpermissive figures, affectionately stern, constraining but consistent. The parent's rigidity reflects clear-cut social sanctions. The grandfather exercises a tender and delicate discipline toward the child. During the early years, the child spends most of his or her time with mother, grandmother, aunts, and other female cousins. During this period, the grandmother is the child's chief source of affection. The child regards all adults as authority figures. This complex of authority figures systematically, and painstakingly teaches the child blind obeisance to his culture. All adults treat all children with great tenderness and great delicacy.

This then is the Cracker culture, and the question is: How can an understanding of this culture help physicians, nurses, and other hospital specialists to a better understanding of their patient's health problems? As briefly as possible, I will provide a few examples.

In most hospitals, visiting rules and regulations are fairly well adapted to the needs of the launching-pad family. Any extended family system, including the Cracker family, is not well served by these arrangements. As one would expect, the Cracker tends to visit the hospital in carloads, particularly when the hospitalized member is in critical condition. It has been my observation that hospital staff find the characteristic visiting practices of extended families difficult to tolerate, and unless the circumstances are extraordinary, family members are dribbled to the patient's bedside in a manner that seems appropriate to a launching-pad family. There is a space problem, but the Cracker patient does feel deprived if his kinsmen are not allowed to cluster in sufficient quantity around his bedside, particularly when he is dying.

[9] This term has gained widespread usage in reference to the consumption patterns of the growing "upper middle class." *See* J. K. Galbraith, *The Affluent Society* (Boston: Houghton Mifflin Company, 1958).

In some instances, the stresses that were eventually responded to by a sickness that required hospitalization would not have been produced in a different culture. A patient with bleeding ulcers provided an excellent example. The patient was a mechanic, and he had been invited into a business partnership by a cousin. The cousin had a country store at a crossroad, and the mechanic moved into an adjacent building to develop a repair shop. The partners had agreed to split the take from both businesses fifty-fifty. The mechanic noticed that his cousin's cash register was fuller on Fridays than it was on Saturdays when the two partners split their take. The mechanic could not question his cousin about this apparent discrepancy without seeming to doubt his trustworthiness. So, the mechanic remained silent, and his cousin continued to appear to cheat him. The mechanic became extremely sick, and he began to feel that he would die if he did not quit the partnership. Without a word to anyone and in the middle of the night he got into his car and set out for Chicago. During the journey he was hospitalized as an emergency case.

The physician understood the Cracker culture. He knew that when a breach between family members cannot be healed, a break with kin and community is made. But, he began to wonder whether the Cracker habit of not openly confronting the offending member when trust seems to have been violated could have resulted in a misunderstanding that was mistaken for untrustworthiness. The physician discovered that this was the case. The mechanic routinely paid for his supplies with cash when he purchased them. The storekeeper ordered his supplies from salesmen who called at the store, and he paid for them by check. The misunderstanding was cleared up. The partnership was mended, and the mechanic's ulcers did not return. The mechanic returned to his family from whom he had been forced to separate himself when he believed that the absolute trust which characterizes the relationships in his culture had broken down.

The Cracker society is a closed society, and as such its members are inhospitable to and distrustful of strangers. This trait can, and sometimes does, make it difficult for hospital specialists to diagnose, treat, and care for patients from this culture. A case in point was a patient who was delivered to the hospital after a car crash. The patient's obvious, and relatively minor, injuries had been sufficiently repaired by the end of the first week, but the physicians were finding it extremely difficult to discover exactly why the patient had lost his ability to speak. For ten days, tests were run and the physicians were still puzzled.

The patient had been insufficiently identified when he was brought to the hospital, and there had been considerable delay in getting information to his family. When the patient had been hospitalized for almost three weeks, several carloads of kin from a distant county came to the hospital to visit him. The staff were amazed when they observed the patient talking freely, and without apparent difficulty, to his kinfolk. Physicians and nurses alike produced elaborate psychological explanations for this interesting phenomenon. Fortunately for their better understanding of the possible importance of cultural factors, one of the surgeons talked to the patient's brother. The surgeon told the brother that the doctors had tried to find out why the patient couldn't talk. The brother replied: "Joe wasn't about to talk. He don't like strangers."

15

Society Invites New Directions

When we think of the changing hospital and the society that produced it as interrelated parts of a complex whole, we can begin to see the direction in which society seems to be inviting the health professions to move. In this chapter, we will examine this invitation.

In our society we have two health systems. A public system chartered to protect society from health hazards, and a private system available to those who are willing and able to seek medical help and to pay for it. These two systems meet in hospitals and clinics where their separate patient-populations are served by the same facilities. Both systems are under pressure to change, and it has become increasingly obvious that society is dissatisfied with the way in which the health professions are organized to distribute diagnosis, treatment, and care.

This dissatisfaction is shared by those in the health professions, and it springs from a growing awareness of the gap between our ability to solve health problems and our actual performance. As far as the health professions are concerned, their suspicion that all is not as good as it could be is confirmed by such things as the international statistics race. For example, despite our unrivaled technology, we have sunk to seventeenth place in our ability to prevent infant mortality.[1] As far as the general public is concerned, this growing awareness is focused on the health systems themselves. The public health system is being criticized for its problem-solving method, and the private health system is under fire because some of its clients feel that they no longer receive the health care they need. These dissatisfactions are somewhat different, and they must be examined separately.

Health workers are problem solvers. They find it difficult to tolerate the knowledge that they are failing to solve as many problems as they are capable of solving. Society seems to them to be suggesting that the private health system should be taken over by the government and administered by bureaucrats. They fear the dead hand of bureaucracy; the fear is not unfounded. Socialized medicine, as it has been developed in other countries, redistributes the supply of diagnosis, treatment, and care at the cost of a cumbersome administrative system which tends to impede the very process it was organized to facilitate. A nation-wide health system in which the decision-making process is centralized near the top of a bureaucratic pyramid would be out of tune with our changing society; that is, this form of organization is becoming obsolete.

Society is dissatisfied with the private health system's delivery practices. The suggestion that socialized medicine is the answer puts the cart before the horse by deciding how health should be paid for before a system capable of delivering the desired level of health has been designed. Complexity as well as cost separate those who wish to use the private health system from the services it provides. The question is how can medical help be made readily available to those who need it? A mere change in payment plan cannot produce an entirely satisfactory solution.

Increasing specialization and a rapidly developing technology have made the private health system both complex and expensive. As far as the potential patient is concerned, cost and complexity combine to increase the distance between the initial appearance of a need for help and the eventual meeting of that need. From the patient's point of view the private health system functions in the following manner. Each member of the family may have his own physician, and each time he seeks cure he may need to seek it from a differently specialized physician. When he finally finds his disease-specific physician, various parts of the diagnostic and treatment process may be parceled out to other specialists. When the patient is able to reach his disease-specific physician without undue delay, the system is satisfactory.

Those who use the private health system value health, and they do not

[1] When I first began to observe the hospital culture, the infant mortality rate in the United States was the third lowest in the world.

begrudge the sacrifices that *must* be made to pay for it. They become distressed when they do not know to whom they should turn. They begrudge the time consumed, the distances covered, and the money spent *before* they reach the specialists who eventually solve their problems. Those who use the private health system value the specialized services it provides. They do not object to paying for these services, and with the exception of two periods during the life cycle, the early child-rearing years and old age, they are in a position to do so. Those who use the private health system need to have its services made more readily available to them. They also need assistance during the two periods when they tend to become "medically indigent."

The medical profession has made and is making various attempts to solve this problem. One approach is to produce a contemporary version of the old-fashioned family doctor. Another is to assemble groups of variously specialized physicians into more or less loosely organized joint practice systems. In addition, the possibility of developing a subphysician category is being explored.

Some medical schools encourage their students to become general practitioners. These attempts have not been entirely successful. Highly specialized professors unwittingly encourage medical students to become specialists. Those who graduate with the intention of practicing family medicine tend to limit their practice to a specialized area after short stints as general practitioners. The "family doctor" has virtually disappeared, and attempts to recreate him as a new speciality do not seem particularly successful. It is safe to say that he has been replaced by an expanding collection of variously specialized physicians.

The subphysician notion is not new. It has been used for a number of years in Russia, and it is being used in countries with critical physician shortages. It may well be that a supply of subphysicians would be useful. The question is: does the private health system need an additional resource, or does it need to use existing resources in a somewhat different manner? To this observer, the primary problem seems to be a traffic problem. Those who use the private health system need to be steered toward the appropriate disease-specific specialist without undue delay. It may be that the "subphysician" could be both a first-aid expert and a traffic expediter.

The third approach, grouping specialized physicians, is not new. Medical specialists were grouped in offices on the same street or in the same building in large cities in western societies before the turn of the present century. Group practice, a formal partnership of differently specialized physicians, ceased to be a novelty in this country during the twenties. Grouping an adequate collection of differently specialized physicians in adjacent offices, and developing a system that would permit the patient to be shunted rapidly to the appropriate specialist or specialists has obvious merit. The "family doctor" has already been displaced as far as urban portions of our population are concerned, but there is no reason why groups of doctors could not practice family medicine. It seems to me that the private health system, in its attempts to make diagnosis and treatment more readily available to its clients, is moving toward the concept of neighborhood health centers. These centers could be made as accessible as shopping centers, and they could develop mechanisms that would move patients rapidly to an appropriate specialist.

It may be that the public health system will move in a similar direction in order to answer a somewhat different criticism. The public health system's problem-solving method is being questioned. This particular criticism is not focused on the public health system. It is a criticism of our society's traditional approach to the problems of those whom we now call "the underprivileged." At the beginning of this century, we were attempting to impose middle-class values on the working classes, and our health and welfare systems reflected this attitude. At the present time, we are working on the assumption that you cannot help anyone unless they want to be helped. This means giving those who need help choices, and encouraging them to become cooperating members of the helping team. The generalized criticism of our traditional "missionary" approach was formalized, as far as the underprivileged in our own country were concerned, when the War on Poverty by-passed the existing welfare structure in order to develop programs in which attempts are made to incorporate the client into the decision-making process.[2]

It is unlikely that the present public health system will be side-stepped in a similar manner, and for the same reason. It is safe to say, however, that the public health system will be under increasing pressure to change its practices in this direction. Society's suggestion seems sensible. As far as this observer is concerned, it is quite obvious that the public health nurse as well as the social worker tends to elicit the Sunday-bill-collector response.[3] Officials of both agencies are sanctioned to coerce and they frequently are treated by their clients as representatives of a hostile status quo. This response creates unproductive therapist-client relationships, and makes it difficult for the public health system to promote the health and well being of its clients. Neighborhood health centers might provide an environment in which a cooperative relationship between the client, and the public health worker could be developed.

[2] B. Davies, "The Jolt to U.S. Social Work." *New Society* (May 25, 1967).

[3] Until relatively recently, the Sabbath was observed, in part, by refraining from dunning people about their debts. When the bill collector first appeared on Sundays, it seemed a monstrous intrusion. Thus, Sunday-bill-collector became a label for a person who is unwelcome, but cannot be forbidden to enter.

The two health systems overlap in the hospital; and, as we have seen, the hospital continues to attempt to impose the patient-role that it originally designed for the indigent and the dying. The traditional patient-role contains contradictory characteristics, and this makes it difficult for patients to sustain it. In addition, it does not permit the sick person to actively cooperate in his own treatment and care. The contradictions in the role make it difficult for the cooperative patient to seem sufficiently submissive. And they make it extremely difficult for the naturally submissive patient to accept abrupt discharge. The traditional patient-role is obsolete, and it is not necessarily therapeutic. Consequently, the hospital is under pressure to change its practice of arbitrarily imposing the traditional patient-role on hospital patients.

Society seems to be inviting its health systems to move in three directions. It is asking that the services of the private health system be made more accessible to those who use these services. It is saying that the public health system's problem-solving method is outmoded. And it is expressing concern about a new category of indigent persons, the medically indigent. During two phases in the life cycle, those who are not otherwise indigent tend to become medically indigent, during the early child-rearing years and after retirement. These are periods during which income tends to be low, and medical expenses tend to be high. Medicare has provided an answer to the second period of medical indigency, but the first period, the early child-rearing years, has not been satisfactorily dealt with.

The question is: How can our two health systems reorganize themselves to deliver the health that their knowledge and technology is capable of producing? How can the health professions rearrange matters so that they can solve all the problems which they now know how to solve? In this section, we will explore some of the possibilities; but, before we do so, we will examine the practical implications of the way in which our society is changing its organizational style. Our society is in the process of redistributing its decision-making rights, and it is obvious that the change from centralized to decentralized decision-making must be taken into account. In order to take cognizance of this significant shift, we must understand it for what it is.

How has industrial man responded to two contradictory concepts, the notion of democracy and the submachine role? For a number of years intellectuals in western societies have been pessimistic about industrial man's ability to survive. This pessimism springs, in part, from a growing awareness of what Weber recognized when he wondered whether it would be possible "to keep a portion of mankind free from the parceling out of the soul, from this supreme mastery of the bureaucratic way of life."

In the beginning it may have been thought that the working classes, for whom the submachine role was designed, would become sufficiently edified to up-date their machine role by using their right to vote. At a time when it was customary to talk about "edifying" the poor and the working classes, vigorous attempts were being made to impose three middle-class virtues, thrift, prudence, and productivity. These virtues were the desired edifications. As Weber [4] saw, however, the organizational system designed to impose the submachine role on those who worked shoulder to shoulder with machines insisted on imposing a similar role on those who worked with paper. The right to vote has not directly interfered with the bureaucratic system's ability to disenfranchise those who work for it. But, the heady notion that all men are born free and to equal opportunity has encouraged industrial man to resist the "parceling-out of the soul" upon which the bureaucratic way of life seems to insist.

In our own brief examination of the changing hospital and the society that has produced it, we have seen, in microcosm, industrial man's resistance to the submachine role. We have seen how this characteristic resistance has created pressures within the society that are gradually reversing society's decision to rob man of the right to make decisions during the working day. We have seen how the bureaucratic form of organization was gradually adopted by most of the large-scale organizations in our society, including our people-processing plants. And we saw how the tide turned, and began to reverse itself as soon as it had become a society of which it could be said that never had so few made decisions for so many. The consequence to the individual of this creeping centralization has made some experts doubt our ability to survive as a society. The reversal of this process should encourage those who have been somewhat pessimistic.

The way in which this reversal was initiated has practical implications for tomorrow's health team. Man sometimes seems a contrary creature, and his response to the elegant logic of rational organization is an excellent example of this apparent contrariness. It is also an excellent example of man's ability to survive. Apparently, man has refused to let his soul be entirely "parceled out by the bureaucratic way of life." We saw how a need to retain a sense of self-determination produced informal action at the lowest level in the bureaucratic pyramid that protected those at these levels from the least tolerable demands of the system. We saw how rational systems eventually stumbled into solutions for the problems created by this protective action. And we discovered that these solutions are similar in one respect: they decentralize decision-making. An important signpost to those responsible for redesigning our health systems, and an interesting comment on the notion that those who are prepared to steal sheep in order to survive would be willing to act like sheep when their food supply has been assured.

As far as industrial societies are concerned, man has given notice that

---

[4] Max Weber, *The Theory of Social and Economic Organization,* A. M. Henderson and T. Parsons, trans. (New York: The Free Press, 1947).

he is not prepared to become a sheep. As a consequence, the right to make decisions is being redistributed to functional levels in America and in other industrial societies. Those who make these changes do not necessarily realize that the innovations they introduce have the potential to change decision-making patterns. Industry was searching for solutions to chronic motivation problems. Prisons shifted their emphasis from punishment to rehabilitation, and in doing so they began to permit decision-making at the lowest level in the system. Mental hospitals introduced the notion of the therapeutic community and began to incorporate those at lower levels in their hierarchies into the decision-making process. In hospitals, the tendency to mimic big business has introduced innovations that have begun to decentralize decision-making. The War on Poverty by-passed the existing welfare structure in order to establish programs that are designed to make the client an actively cooperating member of the team that has been organized to help him. In American society, all social systems are gradually making this type of change. During this same period, the father's absolute right to make decisions for the family has been considerably eroded by new theories about rearing children and managing families.

As far as the health professions are concerned, this significant change has practical implications that cannot be ignored. The decision-making patterns of the systems and institutions designed to produce diagnosis, treatment, and care are changing in such a way as to increase the sense of self-determination of those at lower levels in the hierarchies. This change demands new supervision patterns, new communication patterns, a different style of leadership, and new roles and relationships. In addition, and perhaps most important, it is quite obvious that a health system designed to centralize decision-making toward the top of a bureaucratic pyramid is quite out of the question however laudable its intentions might be. The way in which our society is organized to confront sickness, and to produce health leaves something to be desired; but any modifications we attempt must be in tune with our times. We cannot afford to remake outmoded mistakes.

When we move out of the hospital to confront sickness in its natural habitat, the community, we find two health systems: the public system and a private one. The public health system is paid for out of the public purse, and its primary purpose is to protect society. The private system provides a complete range of services for those who wish to take advantage of it, and are prepared to pay for the services it offers. Until recently, this arrangement was considered satisfactory to society. As we have seen, society and those in the health professions have become increasingly dissatisfied with the delivery of diagnosis and treatment and with the production of health.

In this chapter, we are going to examine some of the factors which might be taken into consideration if we were to attempt to develop a new way of organizing our approach to health. We will begin by considering how the relationships between various members of the health team might be put to productive use. As we shall see, the physician is at some disadvantage when it comes to designing programs to promote health, whereas the nurse and others who have inherited the social distances which characterize the care-role have an initial advantage.

The physician diagnoses the disease, and decides what is to be done about it. He maintains social distance between himself and the patient, and he uses ritual. The physician uses social distance and ritual to establish authority over the disease. The physician waits for the sick person to approach and he scrupulously avoids seeming to solicit his client. By tradition, the phyhician deals with sickness, and in most societies he is paid for attempting cure.[5] It is obvious that the physician is at some disadvantage when it becomes necessary to design preventive programs. Unless a threat to society, such as communicable disease, is being fought, the patient must approach the physician of his own accord; and until the patient is aware of a health problem, he is unlikely to do so. As far as the physician is concerned, the question is: How can those who consider themselves well be encouraged to seek help?

Those roles which derive their characteristics from the care-role, on the other hand, have inherited social distances and a functional style that make it as natural for them to prevent sicknesses as it is for them to care for the sick. In our society, the nurse and the social worker have inherited the social characteristics of their roles from the care-role. The professions that have developed from further specialization of these two professions also are legitimate descendants of the care-role. Traditional usages permit the person in the care-role to offer help and advice even when those being helped do not realize that they need it. As far as the sick are concerned, it is appropriate for the person in the care-role, in our society the nurse, to approach even when the diseases being fought are not considered a threat to society.

The care-role is a wise-sister role: a person who comes to one's aid and to whom one turns in times of trouble. In all societies the wise-sister is a troubleshooter. She comes without undue ceremony when she is informed about trouble, and it is appropriate for her to come without being summoned. Tradition places those in the care-role in intimate relationship with the problems that they are sanctioned to confront. This position gives them tremendous strategic advantages. It also places them in unique

---

[5] An interesting exception was developed in China. Under one traditional system, those who used a cure-specialist on a regular, rather than an emergency basis, paid him as long as they remained in good health. Payments ceased during periods of sickness (personal observation).

jeopardy. Our literature contains numerous examples of women who have used the wise-sister role to become notorious busybodies. Caplan in his book, *An Approach to Community Mental Health*,[6] recognizes that the nurse's unique closeness makes her an effective mental health worker. He does not mention that other helping professions have inherited these social distances.

This inheritance is not always recognized, and in some cases those who inherited the care-role have professionalized themselves by assuming the social characteristics of the cure-role. Some social workers seem to be moving in this direction. When social work emerged as a separate discipline, those who became social workers adopted the social distances and the functional style of the wise-sister role. The unique closeness of that role was obscured by class differences and by society's attempts to impose a middle-class value system on the working classes. Since that time, the professional social worker has begun to assume cure-role characteristics, and she sometimes finds it difficult to offer help when it has not been asked for. This change is due, in part, to an attempt to avoid imposing missionary-style help and, in part, to the notion that people cannot be helped unless they recognize their need for help. These excellent reasons prevent the trained social worker from becoming a busybody, but they make it difficult for her to make help readily available to those who may need it.

I am going to describe a phenomenon which I have observed between 1964 and 1968 that suggests one way in which professional health workers can use the social distances, and the functional style that characterize the care-role to develop productive health-promoting programs. I call this particular phenomenon group-care. In group-care, a professional person becomes health adviser and medical resource expediter to a group of families by becoming a resource person to a number of mothers who have formed themselves into a mutually supportive, information-seeking group. These groups meet at regular intervals to discuss child-rearing and other family problems.

This grouping behavior is characteristic of "middle-class" American mothers, particularly during their child-rearing years. These young women are full-fledged members of the launching-pad society. They practice scientifically determined child-rearing. They are separated from the traditional support of older and more experienced women. And they tend to cluster into groups for mutual support and to seek information.

If, and when, a nurse, a social worker, or a psychologist is available as a resource person, these groups use this person as a consultant about health problems, as an expediter of medical resources, and as a bridge to information from other pertinent disciplines. The young mothers take the

[6] G. Caplan, *An Approach to Community Mental Health* (New York: Grune & Stratton, Inc., 1961).

initiative by forming groups. Through these groups the professional helper becomes the person to whom groups of families turn for help, advice and support. This arrangement places the professional helper in a contemporary version of the wise-sister role. And it permits those in the health field to develop effective and extremely economic health-promoting programs.

There are two impediments to this approach. In some cases, the professional health worker is not entirely sure that group-care is a professional activity. Nurses tend to fall into this category; they enjoy working in this manner, but they are not sure whether or not it is nursing. In other cases, characteristics borrowed from the cure-role inhibit the ability to provide help unless it is formally requested. Psychologists and social workers are sometimes plagued by this particular problem. These difficulties can be surmounted, and the group-care approach appears to have merit.

When I told the nurse [7] around whom such a health-promoting program had developed that I intended to include a description of her program in this book, she was pleased. She was pleased because I recognized what she had done as nursing, but she raised an important issue. She said: "It will take a long time and many articles before other nurses are prepared to recognize that what I am doing is nursing. Until I receive this recognition, I will continue to feel as if what you call nursing, and what I believe is nursing, is merely something I do because I enjoy doing it. At the present moment, it is my hobby, and I cannot *act* as if it is my proper work as a nurse." The young mothers who benefit from this nurse's "hobby" are absolutely convinced that they are the recipients of a most superior brand of nursing.

A response like this is both interesting and disquieting. This particular nurse has explored an extremely productive approach to a major problem. In her spare time, and as a hobby, one nurse has been a catalyst around whom a most promising program has developed. The groups of families who have taken advantage of this program are enthusiastic. The other professional people who have become involved do not doubt either its promise or its professionalism. But, the nurse wonders whether her colleagues will recognize her "hobby" as "work."

There are a number of reasons why this nurse should have responded in this manner. Two of these reasons are interesting and pertinent comments on our culture and on the nursing subculture. This nurse enjoys what she is doing. Nurses, and others in our culture, have been conditioned to suspect the validity of work that seems to be pleasure, a gloomy hangover from a Puritan life style. This nurse does not have scientific proof that what she has accomplished is valid. In recent years, nurses have been asked to prove themselves. As a consequence, they have

[7] Professor Hilliard, College of Nursing, University of Florida.

plunged into the "experiment." This particular nurse was caught unaware. She responded to a demand and an opportunity, and she did not pause to set up variables, instruments, and measures. She merely met a need, and she did so in a creative manner.

This nurse's predicament is not unique. It is the nursing profession's contemporary dilemma. Nurses know that they render a unique service, in many cases against heavy odds. They find it difficult to explain how seemingly unremarkable actions, bathing, feeding, and mere listening, become significant. They are not sure whether their discipline is an art or a science. And they would like to satisfy themselves and society that the small miracles they achieve are based on scientific principles rather than intuitive action. Nursing has been caught in the backlash of the engineering imagination.

Since the beginning of the Industrial Revolution, the intellectual climate of western societies has been dominated by the engineering imagination. The submachine role is an excellent example of the concepts that the engineering imagination characteristically produces when it attempts to deal with social problems.[8] The engineering imagination has produced tremendous technological advances, but its engineering of men has been somewhat less successful than its engineering of matter. The consequence has been the accumulation of problems that require social imagination if they are to be solved.[9] Industrial societies have now become barnacled with social problems. Social problems resist the logic that has permitted western man to master his physical environment. During the past decade, the social imagination has begun to dominate the intellectual climate of western societies. It is ironic that the nurse who functions best when she uses social imagination should feel uneasy because she cannot always produce engineering proofs.

Let me describe how the case in point began. It is a group-care program that may not be recognized as creative nursing. The nurse around whom the group-care program began to develop took turns with other nurses in presenting *Parent's Classes* for expectant parents. At the end of one series of these classes, a young mother in the class asked the nurse to become a resource person to a group of breast-feeding mothers. The nurse agreed, and the relationship between this group of mothers and this particular nurse was extremely productive. Other groups of young mothers and other potential groups heard about this resource nurse. These people sought a similar arrangement. When this happened, the originating mother and the original nurse conceived the notion of meeting this expressed need

[8] The term "engineering imagination" was taken from C. W. Mills, *The Sociological Imagination* (New York: Oxford University Press, 1959).

[9] For a detailed description, read what C. W. Mills refers to as sociological imagination (Mills 1959).

by coordinating clusters of groups in the community around a pool of resource people at a medical center.

At the present moment, there are groups of mothers with children at various age levels and groups of parents with singular problems. The age-level groups fall into such categories as infants, toddlers, grade school, adolescents, and so forth. The singular-problem groups include foreign students, breast feeding, twins, and so forth. The permanent resource pool includes three nurses, a family life expert, two psychologists, a nursing school teacher, an anthropologist, and several members at large who have contributed in various ways to the development of this program.

These groups and this resource pool function in the following manner. Each group has one resource person, in some cases, a nurse and in other cases, another category of professional helper, who informally advises the mothers in the group about child-rearing and other health related problems. This specialist acts as a bridge to the resources of the medical center, the university, and the community. Some groups meet once a week, some twice a month, and others once a month; the resource person sits in with a group, and helps its members to find ways to meet their special needs. In addition to individual groups, there is a coordinating group made up of the chairmen of all groups. The coordinating group meets every three or four months, as the need arises, to coordinate the activities of the groups, to share information, and to decide how the ideas generated by the Environmental Resource Seminar can be implemented.

The Environmental Resource Seminar is made up of permanent resource people, the chairmen of the groups, and members at large. This group meets once a month, and its members take turns presenting a wide range of topics for discussion. This group is particularly interested in discovering what women can do with the resources available to them in American society. In addition to its work with the subsidiary groups, it initiates programs that will enable women to make productive use of existing opportunities. One such program is concerned with designing and initiating part-time jobs to fit the needs of child-rearing women.[10]

The formation of information-seeking, mutually supportive groups during child-rearing is characteristic behavior among "middle-class" women in American society. The way in which these groupings of women used an available nurse and accepted help from other categories of specialists suggested the possibility of trying the same approach in other segments of our society. During the summer of 1966, two graduate students in nursing attempted to capitalize on the natural groupings of child-rearing women

[10] A study of the groups described here was done by G. K. Neville (1965–1967), and the results are reported in G. K. Neville, *The Structure and Function of Child-rearing Study Groups* (M.A. thesis, University of Florida, 1968).

on the porches and at the street-side in a lower socioeconomic community. They secured entry by working with mothers from this community during childbirth. After mother and infant had left the hospital, the students would visit to see the baby. They did not go in a "police" capacity, and they made themselves available by stopping to talk. They found that the women in the community grouped around them, used them as health advisers, and asked them to return. This invitation was accepted and the weekly "visits" of the two students turned into a productive health-promoting program.

This particular venture was interesting because these same women responded in an entirely different manner to two traditional approaches. The public health nurse who served this community routinely elicited the Sunday-bill-collector response. The Red Cross was offering a child-rearing program to this same community during the summer of 1966, and the only people who took advantage of it were two couples from a neighborhood "middle-class" development.

Grouping around a nurse seems to be a characteristic of child-rearing women in our society, and I had observed this phenomenon a number of times before I realized the significance of what I was observing. A nurse triggers behavior like this from those who live in her neighborhood. The attendance patterns at laundromats shifted when the clientele become aware of the fact that a nurse routinely does her wash at a specific time during the week. At PTA meetings, at church gatherings, and at other formal meetings a nurse invariably attracts grouping behavior. In the numerous instances of this phenomenon that I have observed, the group seeks to use the nurse as a health adviser and as a bridge to specialized information and resources. Other categories of health-related specialists trigger this grouping behavior, and are used in a similar manner if they are willing to help others on an informal basis. It is not considered "professional" to deliver "back fence" health care. Consequently this phenomenon is discouraged rather than capitalized.

The group-care program described in this chapter has been developed by making opportunistic use of the natural grouping behavior of child-rearing women. This phenomenon is not limited to child-rearing women. In our society there is a general tendency to group around common activities and problems. Physicians, nurses, and other applied disciplines hold periodic meetings. Bell ringers, writers, and other artists gather into formal groups in a similar manner. Undertakers and housekeepers attend annual meetings. In a somewhat similar way, people with common problems group for support and to exchange information. The nurse and others who have inherited the social distances that characterize the wise-sister role could capitalize on this phenomenon, and act as advisors to groups of diabetics, to colostomy clubs, and to other natural clusterings of those with common health problems. The psychiatric social worker could use this approach to develop mental health programs. Both the psychologist and the nurse could promote effective child-rearing in a similar manner. It seems to me that the health professions might make opportunistic use of natural grouping behavior to develop effective and economical health-promoting programs in all segments of our society.

This approach could be used by the public health system to update its problem-solving method. A new trend in public health thinking has begun to emerge, and this new thinking seems to be moving in this general direction. In some schools the public health nurse is being taught to begin by characterizing the social structure of the community. An understanding of the dynamics of a particular community are then used by the student to identify its health problems, and to develop solutions that make use of, rather than run counter to, community dynamics.

16

*Bridging the Gap
between Hospital
and Community*

The group-care program described in the last chapter could be organized into the health system in a number of different ways. It could be based in the Public Health Department or in the local hospital. It could be community sponsored and function out of city hall. It could be based in a neighborhood health center, and it could be offered by a local physician as a public service. In this chapter, we will examine the possibility of basing it in the hospital, and of allowing it to serve an additional purpose: bridging the gap between the hospital and the community.

The hospital is decentralizing its decision-making to functional levels, and this change demands new supervision patterns and a new style of leadership. These demands most visibly affect two offices: the Hospital Administrator's Office and the Nursing Service Office. We will examine the possibility of making use of the changing functional style of these two offices to develop group-care programs. We will begin by examining the changing function of the Nursing Service Office, and see if we might use existing resources to provide this additional service. Then we will consider various ways in which the hospital administrator could cooperate to make the group-care program a bridge between the hospital and the community.

The traditional functions of the Nursing Service Office are to administer the nursing services that are provided in the hospital, and to act as a communication channel with other parts of the system. The person who occupies this office is used by others in the system in interesting ways. The director of Nursing Service is the primary scapegoat in the traditional hospital culture. She or he is used for this purpose by the hospital administrator, by the various department heads, and by the chiefs of services. The person in this office also is used as a source of medical information on which administrative decisions are based. In addition, the person in this office is expected to see to it that the hospital continues to discharge its responsibilities to and for the patient-population when other categories of hospital specialists are no longer on the premises.

The uses to which the person in this office are put has produced patterns of supervision and a style of leadership that become obsolete as soon as an administrative arm is extended into the patient-care units. Even in those cases in which the lay managers of the units are responsible to the Nursing Service Office, these obsolescences become visible. Nurses sometimes refer to the traditional supervision style that they use as "snoopervision."

The snooper element tends to be present in any supervision style that develops in systems organized to centralize decision-making. In these systems those who supervise are supposed to see to it that those beneath them in the hierarchy do what they have been told to do in exactly the way that they have been told to do it. The supervised use their informal social system to see to it that they are not caught cutting corners. It is interesting to watch the changes in activity that *precede* a supervisor as he or she moves around the premises. It is like Catherine the Great's trip from Moscow to the Black Sea. Catherine the Great had grandiose notions about developing the interior of Russia. She caused a road to be planned from Moscow to the Black Sea, and ordered a population to flank the road. From time to time she received progress reports. One day she decided to see for herself. This decision precipitated an historical hoax. The road was made as Catherine was being trundled majestically along it. And the distant towns and villages that were pointed out to her were silhouettes that were assembled, dismantled, and reassembled at appropriate intervals.[1] In a similar manner, the appearance of work as it has been ordered to be done is fabricated during the nursing supervisor's inspections.

The classical snooper element is present in traditional nursing supervision. In addition, the nursing supervisor is expected to "snoop out"

[1] From Marquis de Cusine, *Journey For Our Time,* P. P. Kohler, ed. and trans. (New York: Farrar, Straus & Giroux, Inc., 1951).

items of information that will permit the director of Nursing Service to provide the hospital administrator with sufficient understanding to make administrative decisions that directly affect the working situation of individual physicians. When lay managers are introduced at the patient-care unit level, this second snooper element is no longer necessary. The unit manager has the required information, and passes it directly to the office to which he or she is responsible. If the unit manager is responsible to the Nursing Service Office, the director of Nursing Service continues to provide the hospital administrator with this information, but the nursing supervisor is by-passed in the process. When the unit manager is responsible to the Administrator's Office the nursing supervisor and the director of Nursing Service are by-passed.

In an unpublished paper P. Laurencelle described the change in response to traditional nursing supervision when a lay manager was introduced at the patient-care unit level. The nurses in charge of the patient-care units were no longer able to tolerate traditional supervision. The supervisor did not have the authority over the nurse in charge that she had previously had over the head nurses, and she no longer rendered a service. One of the functions of the traditional nursing supervisor is to facilitate services and supplies. This function had been assumed by the units' lay managers. The introduction of a lay management system on patient-care units makes the offices of the night and evening supervisors redundant, and it demands new patterns of supervision and leadership from those who function out of the Nursing Service Office.

When decentralized management is used in nursing services, the nurses in the hospital continue to need support and leadership. They cease to need traditional supervision from the Nursing Service Office, and they find it difficult to tolerate such supervision when the supervisor no longer is able to reward and punish them by manipulating hospital services and supplies. The Nursing Service Office retains its primary reward system— promotion and other recognitions of excellent performance—and loses a system of rewards and punishments that it frequently used unwittingly.

When decentralized management is used, it becomes necessary to decide what kind of support, leadership, and supervision would be most productive. The object of the exercise is to produce quality patient-care as economically as possible, and the nurse's function is to see to it that this product is delivered to the patient. The question is: What can the Nursing Service Office provide that will enable the nurse to deliver quality patient-care?

Quality patient-care must be defined and a criteria suggested. Dorothy M. Smith[2] suggests one way in which it can be defined. Industry defines quality by specifying it, and customarily guarantees to deliver its product

[2] Conversation with Dean Smith, College of Nursing, University of Florida, 1963.

according to these specifications. Nursing could use a similar approach. The basic needs of *all* patients could be identified, and the action required to meet these needs could be specified. All patients need to be clean, safe, and as comfortable as possible. What action must be taken by the nurse to provide these specified components of patient-care? What additional action must be taken under the various special circumstances that characteristically apply to different segments of the hospital's patient-population? The treatment plan of all patients must be implemented. Changes in each patient's condition must be detected and appropriate action based on these changes initiated. The integrity of the therapeutic environment must be maintained. Defining quality patient-care requires detailed specification about what action must be taken if these and other components of patient-care are to be produced.

Delivering the patient-care specified requires action by the nurse. Her action may bring her into direct contact with the patient. It may cause another person to do something for the patient; it may mobilize a resource on the patient's behalf, or it may be a pertinent communication about the patient. The nurse organizes patient-care, and she mobilizes the resources to deliver it. In some cases she plans it, in other cases she sees to it that the physician's plans for the treatment of the patient are carried out, and in other cases routine hospital practices set limits within which patient-care must be planned.

The Nursing Service Office provides the leadership and support that will enable the nurse to describe and deliver quality patient-care. And the Nursing Service Office supervises this process. It recognizes productive innovations, and it discourages unproductive practices. The Nursing Service Office sees to it that adequate levels of patient-care are established and maintained. This important function demands two distances: an intimate involvement with concrete patient-care problems and a distance that provides perspective, and keeps the problems of each unit in institutional perspective.

This supportive supervision could be provided by rejuvenating the jaded notion of a "float team."[3] The director of Nursing Service could become a facilitator of quality patient-care, and this function could be supported by transforming the traditional hierarchy of supervisors into a team of clinical specialists with three primary functions. Their schedules would be flexible. They would work where most needed either because of staff shortages or because the staff had recognized a problem that they, themselves were unable to solve without assistance. Approaching in this manner would earn the kind of welcome rarely accorded to traditional supervisors. Whenever a clinical specialist was pinch-hitting in this manner,

[3] The "float team" traditionally fills gaps. Members of it are assigned on an *ad hoc* basis to those units that are short of staff on any particular shift.

she would be rendering two additional services. She would be providing In-Service Education by teaching those with whom she was working to become more effective clinicians. And she would be gathering first-hand experiences that would permit her to develop practical solutions to chronic problems. She would become a working consultant and teacher in her own clinical speciality. In addition, she could become a bridge between clinical specialities. The psychiatric nurse, for example, has skills and knowledge that could be applied to other nursing specialities. Backed up by this team, the director of Nursing Service could provide the supportive supervision that the contemporary situation seems to demand.

Once this team of clinical specialists had been established, it could expand its function to include the development of a group-care program similar to the one described in the last chapter. Such a program does not demand excessive amounts of time, a few hours a month, or, at most, a few hours a week would be all that one nurse would be asked to contribute. Both the hospital and the patient would profit by this program out of all proportion to the time expended. The hospital is inadequately linked with the community, and this inadequacy produces two faults in the health system. The hospital is not sufficiently supported by community resources. And the patient tends to be returned to the community with insufficient therapeutic supports. A group-care program based in the Nursing Service Office could be used to correct these two faults.

It is extremely discouraging to hospital workers when a patient deteriorates after he has been released from the hospital merely because the hospital has no mechanism through which its workers can help the family to provide the continuing care that the former patient requires. The new infant is frequently released to parents who will need advice, but do not know to whom they should turn for advice during the first weeks of their infant's life. The patient who has partially recovered his former ability to care for himself may deteriorate merely because his family needs advice and reassurance during the first weeks when they are learning how to provide the care needed. In some cases patients like this one are shipped off to scrap institutions. This chronic gap is sometimes closed by referring the patient to the Public Health System, but the public system is neither chartered nor equipped to completely bridge this particular gap. A group-care program firmly linked to the hospital's resources would provide a less cumbersome and more effective bridge for the former patient.

The new patient needs a bridge. To most patients the hospital is a strange and terrifying place. If through group-care the patient, or a member of his family, were already acquainted with a nurse who was intimately associated with the hospital, the new patient would enter the hospital with less trepidation. Those who worked with the patient in the hospital would have readier access to information about him. Furthermore, it is reasonable to assume that the new patient's hospital experience would be more productive if it were based on a continuing relationship between a nursing clinician and either the patient or some member of his family.

These rearrangements could be achieved without directly involving the hospital administrator. The patient would profit by not being shunted into an entirely alien social situation at a time when he is least capable of coping with the strange and the potentially terrifying. The staff would be less frustrated because they would have information about the patient readily available to them, and because there would be a mechanism through which they could continue to help the patient after he had left the hospital if, and when, this help seemed either desirable or necessary. If the hospital administrator became involved, he could see to it that this patient-care bridge was used to link the hospital to community resources.

The hospital is a resource that affluent communities seem unable to afford. All human societies value health in as much as they value a sense of physical well being. In our society we value health, and we expect it to be expensive to maintain. Although our society sets a high value on the hospital's product, it has not satisfactorily solved the problem of paying for that product. However, the community does recognize an obligation to the hospital, and expresses this obligation by contributing time and money to its support. The precedent on which the hospital administrator could build has been set.

Before we consider possible action, let us examine one of the changes in functional style that seems to be demanded from the hospital administrator when decentralized management is introduced. The primary function of the administrator is to support and facilitate patient-care. Decentralizing decision rights out of his office into a number of other offices turns the administrator from a problem solver into a solution coordinator. Problems are no longer sent to superior offices for solutions, they are solved at functional levels. From his superior office, the administrator surveys the scene spotting problems that have not been recognized as such, encouraging the solution of recognized problems, and providing institutional perspective. In addition, he coordinates the solutions that emerge from all parts of the system.

When his hospital has developed a bridge to the community, the administrator sees this bridge as a mechanism through which services flow out and resources flow in. In the group-care program described in the last chapter, community resources began to move into the medical center in a natural manner, and it was some time before anyone recognized that an exchange was in progress. The relationships between resource persons and group members produced mutual involvement in professional problems. It seemed natural to resource persons to enrich a lecture by inviting a group member to be present as a live case history whom the students could question freely. It seemed natural to group members to suggest innovations in hospital practices. And both the resource person and the group member took it for granted that if the hospital did not have the necessary resources they, the group members, would work together to mobilize these resources from the community. The "How are we going to solve this problem?" response emerged as soon as mutual involvement occurred.

It seems to me that a hospital administrator could use a group-care program to involve the community in hospital problems. Any community, however poverty stricken, has untapped resources, many of which are intangible. As soon as a community begins to personalize an institution, it begins to mobilize time, skills, monies, and other artifacts to provide solutions for institutional problems. When community members begin to think about *our* hospital, they begin to feel responsible for seeing to it that their hospital has the resources it needs to solve its problems. As long as community members continue to think of the hospital as *the* hospital, they discharge their obligations to the institution in a somewhat different manner. They use the hospital's need for volunteers as an opportunity to create elite clubs. They fund raise as a civic gesture, and they donate sums of money that are appropriate to their positions in the community. They use the hospital's needs to endow memorials to themselves. And they express their reluctance to throw away things of possible use by dumping magazines and discarded clothing at the hospital. As long as it remains *the* hospital, the community will not be sufficiently involved to mobilize the resources that a hospital needs in order to solve its problems.

If the hospital and its specialists are to work with the community in the ways suggested in this chapter, they will need a working understanding of social systems and subcultures. At the present moment the health professions teach their students the specialized services they will be expected to deliver, but for the most part, they do not provide students with a sufficient understanding of the subcultures from which their patients will come, and of the social systems within which their attempts to deliver the services they have been taught to provide will be made. This book is an attempt to make social systems and cultural differences visible, and to suggest how physicians, nurses, and other professional health workers might make use of this information.

In Horizontal Orbit would be incomplete without a word about death, and my observations of it suggest that it would be desirable, and might be possible, to bridge the widening gap between the dying and the living. Two books [4] about the dying are recommended as more explicit statements of the implications suggested in the final pages.

[4] B. G. Glaser and A. L. Strauss, *Awareness of Dying* (Chicago: Aldine Publishing Company, 1965); and J. Hinton, *Dying* (Baltimore: Penguin Books, Inc., 1967).

17

A Word about Dying

"Men fear death as children fear to go in the dark; and as that natural fear in children is increased with tales, so is the other." [1] Dread of death makes it difficult for us to speak about death, but it is interesting to talk to people about the death they would choose. Both the dying and the nondying would like to die quickly, as painlessly as possible, and without burdening those close to them. They would like to die with dignity, to go out with a bang rather than a whimper. In a sense society sets the stage on which each of us, at one time or another, will play out this role to its inevitable end, and although we cannot write our own scripts, we can look at the cast of characters that will support us during our final drama.

The role of the physician is to see to it that the play lasts as long as possible, and that the pain which must be endured is muted. The hero can expect the physician to encourage him to hope that the present performance is a dress rehearsal. The physician will be on stage at regular intervals. During the early scenes these appearances will be supplemented

[1] Francis Bacon, *Of Death*.

184

by periodic entrances during which the drama is heightened by vigorous battles with death. During final scenes, the physician confines himself to routine appearances, and the dialogue between the physician and the hero is ritualized. The physician may not be present when the final curtain goes down, but he will be summoned, and he will hasten backstage to certify that the play has, in fact, ended.

The nurse's role is a supportive one. Her task is to see to it that the hero meets death with dignity, and that he is made as comfortable as possible while he is waiting for it. This role is played by a number of different persons, and it is not unusual for more than one of them to be on stage at the same time. This is particularly true in the early phases of the drama when the physician enters to stage battles with death. As the play drags on, the stage becomes less crowded with persons in the nurse's role, and if the hero takes "an unconscionable time adying," [2] he may spend most of the time alone on stage. As the play draws to an end, he will notice that those in the nurse's role bustle on stage at eight-hour intervals seeming to encourage him to stage his final scene during the next shift.

For the most part our hero confronts death in an institution, hospital, or nursing home, and those close to him, family and friends, are allowed access to him according to the rules and regulations of the institution, and according to the discretion of the physician. It is usual practice to keep these actors off stage in specialized waiting areas frequently called "family rooms" where, like "extras" during the production of a movie, they are readily available for walk-on parts and crowd scenes.

Death has become a lonely process, and, for the most part, the scripts of these dramas avoid clear statements about the theme of the play. The physician knows that the hero is dying, but he is not sure when, and he does not want to discourage his patient from hoping that it is a dress rehearsal. Off stage the physician talks to the "extras," family and friends, about "probabilities"; in the wings he talks to those in the nurse's role about "inevitabilities"; and during dialogue with the hero he talks about "possibilities." Thus, the central character in the death drama is told that although it is possible he will die, it also is possible that he may live to die at another time. Those closest to the dying person are told that it is probable that he will die. Those whose role it is to see that he dies with dignity and as comfortably as possible, the nurses, are told that, barring a miracle, death is inevitable. Although from time to time the nurses have seen miracles, the miracle with which they are most familiar is one that pushes the death scene into the next shift.

These four levels of information produce dialogues that are reminiscent of the double dialogues parents attempt when they talk with each other

<hr />

[2] Charles II's classical apology for taking an inordinate time to die.

about young children in their presence. In its simplest form, key words are spelled out; at a more sophisticated level foreign languages are used. Children sometimes turn the tables on adults by inventing "secret" languages, "Pig Latin" is an excellent example. Double dialogues, both on and off stage, in the death drama are more complex than the game adults and children sometimes play with each other, but they are played in the same way. The object of "double dialogue" is to talk about a problem involving someone within earshot without letting him know what you are talking about. Both the child and the dying patient learn to interpret the remarks that are not intended for their ears, but the consequences are somewhat different. The child can make use of the conversation that is supposed to be "above his head" to outwit his parents. The dying person may profit by finding out what he wants to know, but if he needs to talk with others about the fact that he is dying, he will find that "double dialogue" is designed to prevent him from mentioning this matter to anyone except the chaplain.

Like most members of our society, I avoid death, and in my study of the hospital culture, I avoided dying patients for three years and talking about death with them for five. When eventually I forced myself to talk about death with the dying, I discovered a number of things that surprised me:

> I found that I had unwittingly discouraged patients from talking about death. A woman said: "I tried to talk about it with you last week, but like everyone else, you changed the subject." A young man said: "You knew I wanted to hammer it out, but every time I started you remembered something else you had to do."

> I found that those who were dying welcomed an opportunity to talk with a stranger about living and dying. One man said: "I don't want a minister fussing around about my soul, I want a human being to talk to." Another said: "It's like I got bad breath or something—the people around here act as if I shouldn't want to talk about it (death)."

> I found that some patients wanted to know as soon as possible that they were going to die. One man said: "I know she (his wife) acted for the best, but she should have let the doctor tell me six months ago. I needed time to put my affairs in order." And a young mother said: "They (husband and physician) should have told me. I could have prepared the kids and helped my husband."

> I found that hospitals do not always permit the farewell that seems most appropriate to the dying person. A person from the Cracker culture said: "They (the staff) let them in one at a time. If I were at home all my kin would sit up and see me through." An old lady said: "There's no one left but my dog. I visit with him over the phone, but

its not like seeing him to say goodbye." And a young woman said: "Now I can die in peace. They (the nurses) wheeled me out, and I said goodbye. I wish the kids could have come to my room; it was rough on them with strangers hanging around watching and listening."

I found that some patients dreaded not being dead after they had ceased to be alive. One woman said: "My mother was like a vegetable for six months before she died. I can stand the pain, but I pray to be spared that." A man said: "I'm going to will myself dead as soon as I begin to loose grip." Another said: "It violates my sense of human dignity."

I found that the sense of dignity is assured in relatively simple ways. The young woman who took leave of her "kids" in a corridor asked to be "freshened up," thanked the nurses, sent her husband off for a "good night's sleep," closed her eyes and said: "Don't call him until eight; and when you do say that the last thing I said was: thank you for our life together." An old man who had not been out of bed for three weeks said: "Son, get me out of bed while she (the nurse) is out of the way. I want to 'pee' like a man again before I die." When this had been done, he said: "No need to tell her about it just say that I already done it. Goodbye, son. I'm going to sleep and I don't intend to wake."

Some years ago I asked a visitor from India about how death is handled in Indian hospitals, and was told that death rarely occurs in them. "When nothing more can be done, the dying are sent back to their families. When this decision has not been made promptly enough, the families are distressed. In India death is a family affair, and we are upset when members of our family die among strangers." In our society death has ceased to be a family affair, and it is probable that each of us will die among strangers who are reluctant to talk with us about the fact that we are dying. In our society death has become a lonely process.

NOTES

Notes

PART ONE   The Hospital

1.   Relevant Theory: The hospital is a large-scale organization, and a theoretical frame of reference for it should be based on relevant theory about this social system. What I label "the large-scale organization" usually is referred to as a ——— organization, the blank being a delineating adjective, formal, complex, bureaucratic, and so forth. I prefer to lump social systems like this together as "large-scale" in order to suggest an interesting characteristic: they tend to increase in size whether or not this increase is expressed by a comparable increase in productivity. Furthermore, I differentiate them by nouns suggesting function: hospital, prison, factory, and so forth, rather than adjectives describing the way in which they are organized to function. My reason for doing so is twofold. As Weber [1] pointed out and Parsons [2] emphasized, the differentiating characteristic of such systems is that they are organized to accomplish a specific task. Originally, it was assumed that these organizations invariably were, and would be, administered in a bureaucratic manner; an assumption that observations sometimes contradict.

There is a vast amount of literature about the large-scale organization, but the prime shapers of relevant theory are Weber and Barnard. Weber identified the distinguishing characteristic mentioned above (Weber 1947: 151–152). He made other points that were confirmed by my own observations, and provided insights into them. It is a "corporate group" defined as "a social relationship which is either closed or limits the admission of outsiders by rules and will be called a 'corporate group' *(Verband)* so far as its order is enforced by the action of specific individuals whose regular function this is, of a chief or 'head' *(Leiter)* and usually also an administrative staff" (Weber 1947: 145–146). The notion of members and nonmembers and the suggestion that under appropriate circumstances there could be a submembership-by-rule group has been particularly useful. It helps to explain a phenomenon encountered from time to time, the nonmember "passing" as a member. For example, there have been cases of persons, dressed in white coats with stethescopes hanging out of a pocket, who have moved freely about hospitals acting like doctors without being challenged. The hospital admits "outsiders by rules," and one category of person admitted in this manner, the patient, temporarily becomes a member of a closed group, the patient-population. Thus, the hospital contains two closed groups: its staff and its patients. Interestingly enough, it is easier for a nonmem-

---

[1] Max Weber, *The Theory of Social and Economic Organization,* trans. A. M. Henderson and T. Parsons (New York: The Free Press, 1947), pp. 151–152.

[2] T. Parsons, *Structure and Processes in Modern Society* (New York: The Free Press, 1960), p. 17.

ber to "pass" as a member of the staff than as a member of the patient-population, primarily because the nonmember attempting to "pass" as a patient would find it difficult to get the papers needed to support this disguise. Weber's statement that the function of administration is to "enforce the system's order" is ineresting because the administrative syle of the large-scale organization has shifted since I began looking at it thirty years ago. It has shifted from "enforce" to "control" to "coordinate." A look at Barnard's [3] frame of reference suggests why.

Barnard identified the fundamental "elements" of organization as: communication; willingness to contribute; and common purpose (Barnard 1938: 82). Given these elements his conclusion was that the essence of formal organization is the making of decisions. A brilliant insight, and one that has been particularly productive because the most significant change in the large-scale organization during the past thirty years has been a redistribution of decision-making rights and a consequent modification of administrative style that alters a bureaucracy, in some cases changing it into a corporate system. It is interesting that when I began to examine the large-scale organization, I felt that I owed a primary debt to Weber because I patterned my observations of structure and function on his insights. Although I looked at decision-making patterns, as suggested by Barnard, I did not consider them particularly important. They have been most important not only because they alerted me to a significant change in organizational form but also because they drew my attention to the informal system and action that functions to modify the decisions made by the formal system.

In my text, I have presented examples of the "tug-of-war" between the formal and the informal systems, and offered some explanation of it. Others have formulated more explicit models of this interesting battle; and although their terminology differs slightly from mine, the emphasis is the same—that the objectives of the formal and informal systems must be compatible if the organization is to function effectively. The following sources are suggested: P. M. Blau, *Bureaucracy in Modern Society* (New York: Random House, Inc., 1956); Parsons 1960; and P. Selznick, "An Approach to a Theory of Bureaucracy," *Amer. Sociol. Rev.* 13 (1948): 25–35.

The two threads of thought begun by Weber and Barnard can be traced through the literature; but before we do so, it is necessary to add one further point made by Weber which is that an organization *(betriebsverband)* is "associative" rather than "communal" in character (Weber 1947: 136–139). This comment draws our attention to the time and energy spent "manufacturing" social cohesion, a phenomenon that is particularly noticeable in extremely large organizations, and one that leads us to suspect that large-scale organizations find it difficult to remain cohesive enough to function effectively. Parsons, who helped to translate Weber's work, appears to have been influenced by him. He placed major emphasis on Weber's criterion: "it (the organization) is engaged in carrying out continuous purposive, activity of a specified kind (Weber 1947: 151–152), by saying: "Primacy of orientation to the attainment of a specific goal is used as the defining characteristic of an organization which distinguishes

---

[3] C. I. Barnard, *The Function of the Executive* (Cambridge, Mass.: Harvard University Press, 1938).

it from other types of social systems" (Parsons 1960: 17). But Parsons moved toward Barnard in the emphasis he placed on the "shared" and "collective" goals of organizations (T. Parsons and E. A. Shils, eds. *Toward a General Theory of Action* [Cambridge, Mass.: Harvard University Press], 1954, p. 192). Simon follows the trail blazed by Barnard inasmuch as he uses Barnard's decision premise as a central unit of organizational analysis (H. A. Simon, *Administrative Behavior,* 2d ed. [New York: Macmillan, 1957]). Simon's approach, basing his work on one of the two theororists, is more usual than Parsons' approach which is to move from one toward the other. Most usually Weber's and Barnard's theories of organization have been thought of as conflicting. Hopkins shows them, as I have found them in the practical situation, complementary (T. K. Hopkins, "Bureaucratic Authority: the Convergence of Weber and Barnard" in *Complex Organizations,* A. Etzioni, ed. [New York: Holt, Rinehart and Winston, Inc., 1961], pp. 82–98).

There have been some interesting comments about the way in which the large-scale organization emerges in societies with sufficiently developed divisions of labor. Parsons (1960: 14) says: "The development of organizations is the principle mechanism by which, in a highly differentiated society, it is possible to 'get things done,' to achieve goals beyond the individual." Weber made an early attempt to describe the conditions that were required for the emergence of bureaucratic organization, the preferred model in industrial societies until relatively recently.[4] Eisenstadt[5] compares examples in western and nonwestern societies, and suggests that the following conditions encourage the emergence of bureaucratic organization: a high degree of differentiation among roles and industrial spheres; allocation of the crucial roles by universalistic rather than particularistic criteria; extending the boundaries of the community to include more than one particularistic group; increasing complexity of social life; group attempts to develop and pursue common goals (social, economic, political, and so forth) that extend beyond the boundaries of any particularistic group; competition among groups for scarce resources, and the development of different priorities and goals among groups. (Eisenstadt 1958: 110).

There has been a tendency to think of bureaucratic organization as immutable. However, many observers, including myself, have reported contradictions in bureaucratic structures and changes in them. W. Delaney, ("The Development and Decline of Patrimonial Administrations," *Admin. Sci. Quart.* 7 (1963): 458–501) takes cognizance of these modifications, and speaks of emergence of "post-bureaucratic" forms. Interestingly enough, Weber (1947: 68) apparently considered bureaucratic structure less stable than structures supported by traditional relations, and might have predicted the emergence of "post-bucreaucratic" forms.

2. *The Hospital and Its History:* Those interested in the history of the hospital might begin by looking at the first two chapters in *The Hospital in Modern*

---

[4] Max Weber, *From Max Weber: Essays in Sociology,* H. H. Gerth and C. W. Mills, eds. and trans. (New York: Oxford University Press, 1946), pp. 204–214.

[5] S. N. Eisenstadt, "Bureaucracy and Bureaucratization," *Curr. Sociol.* 7 (1958): 99–163.

Society: Eleven Studies of the Hospital Today, E. Freidson, ed. (New York: The Free Press, 1963). The chapter by G. Rosen is "The Hospital: Historical Sociology of a Community Institution" (pp. 1–36), and the one by W. A. Glaser is "American and Foreign Hospitals: Some Sociological Comparisons" (pp. 37–72). Each chapter is supported by notes that are a comprehensive guide to pertinent literature. Two chapters in *Patients, Physicians, and Illness,* E. G. Jaco, ed. (New York: The Free Press, 1958) present theory relevant to discussion about the hospital as a social system: A. B. Wessen's, "Hospital Ideology and Communication between Ward Personnel" (pp. 448–468) and H. L. Smith's, "Two Lines of Authority" (pp. 468–477). Doctors Brown, Caudill, and von Mering and King have made significant contributions to our understanding of the hospital. All three of them present their material in such a way as to make their books both rewarding and delightful reading: E. L. Brown, *Newer Dimensions of Patient Care,* Part 2 (New York: Russell Sage Foundation, 1962); O. von Mering, and S. H. King, *Remotovating The Mental Patient* (New York: Russell Sage Foundation, 1957); and W. Caudill, *The Hospital as a Small Society* (Cambridge, Mass.: Harvard University Press, 1958).

I have found the following two relatively recent books about organizations particularly stimulating: J. K. Galbraith, *The New Industrial State* (Boston: Houghton Mifflin Company, 1967) and A. Jay, *Management and Machiavelli: An Inquiry into the Politics of Corporate Life* (New York: Holt, Rinehart and Winston, Inc., 1968).

Whitehead suggested a frame of reference for hospital roles and relationships when he suggested that during his life cycle an individual "will be called upon to face novel situations which find no parallel in his past. The fixed person for the fixed duties, who, in older societies was such a godsend, in future will be a public danger." (cited in L. H. Evans and G. E. Arnstein, "Automation and Education: Hypothesis for a Partial Answer" [Washington, D.C.: *National Education Association*, January 1962], p. 3). It is obvious that industrial man not only is socialized during childhood but also is resocialized over and over again during the course of a single lifetime. It also is obvious that in a rapidly changing society such as ours, individuals must be prepared for roles about which those who are socializing them can only guess. This concept of socialization and a recognition of the role of rapid change are pertinent to theory about hospital roles and relationships.

1. Hospital Roles and Relationships: As an introduction: H. S. Becker and J. W. Carper, "The Development of Identification with Occupation" (*Amer. J. Sociol.* (1956): 289–298) is recommended. T. R. Williams and M. M. Williams, "The Socialization of the Student Nurse" (*Nursing Res.* 8 (1959); 18–25) is particularly valuable in that it reviews the demands made on the nursing students to modify their attitudes toward death, unpleasant odors, and the exposed human body. S. E. Cleveland, "Personality Patterns Associated with the Professions of Dietitian and Nurse" (*J. Health and Human Behavior* 2 (September 1961): 113–124) helps us to understand the nurse and the dietitian, and suggests why nurses and dietitians seem to be in chronic conflict with each other.

The material by E. C. Hughes "The Making of a Physician" (*Hum. Organ.* 14 (1956): 21–25) and R. K. Merton, G. C. Reader, and P. L. Kendall, *The Student Physician: Introductory Studies in the Sociology of Medical Education* (New York: The Free Press, 1957) serves as an adequate introduction to the unique problem of becoming a physician. Section V "Becoming a Physician: Medical Education" in *Patients, Physicians, and Illness*, E. G. Jaco, ed. (New York: The Free Press, 1958, pp. 288–250) provides an excellent summation of becoming and being a physician.

Many occupational roles in the hospital are thought of as careers; and careers, as the literature suggests, can be separated into stages. D. C. Miller and W. Form, *Industrial Sociology: An Introduction to the Sociology of Work Relations.* (New York: Harper & Row, Publishers, 1951) provides an excellent introduction to this notion by dividing the life cycle into five stages: preparatory (0–15 years), initial work period (15–18 years), trial work period (18–34 years), stable work period (34–64 years), and retirement. O. Hall, "The Stages in a Medical Career" (*Amer. J. Sociol.* 54 (1948): 327–336) identifies and characterizes four stages in a medical career. A similar approach could be used to analyze the careers of other categories of health specialists. Those professsions dominated by female members, nursing, for example, would have to take cognizance of the dropout during child-rearing years and of the way in which middle-aged, "middle-class" American women are invading the labor market. It also should consider specialties like hospital administration in which the road to success tends to be via rapid moves from institution to institution rather than by makng a name for oneself in one institution. Florio's examination of the career patterns of city managers is interesting from this point of view: G. K. Florio, "Continuity in City-Manager Careers" (*Amer. J. Sociol.* 61 (1955): 240–246). H. S. Becker, and A. Strauss, "Careers, Personality, and Adult Socialization" (*Amer. J. Sociol.* 62 (1956): 253–263) can be thought of as summing up career studies.

Another aspect of socialization is pertinent, and that is to think about the way in which organizations socialize subsets of their members. The primary goal of some organizations is to socialize one such subset; prisons and mental hospitals fall into this category. E. Goffman in *Asylums* (New York: Doubleday Anchor, 1961) describes the characteristics of organizations having this primary function, in considerable detail. In other organizations, including general hospitals, the socialization function is secondary, and orientation programs for new employees is a usual expression of it. A. Etzioni in *A Comparative Analysis of Complex Organization* (New York: The Free Press, 1961) discusses socialization as a secondary function. Educating professional health workers and "teaching programs" for hospital and clinic patients are other examples of the socialization function. The way in which those being socialized set limits on formal socialization programs should interest students who are being prepared to become professional health workers. H. S. Becker, B. Greer, E. C. Hughes, and A. L. Strauss, *Boys in White* (Chicago: University of Chicago Press, 1961) is recommended as a beginning reading. For nursing students, an additional reading is suggested: R. G. Corwin, "The Professional Employee: A Study of Conflict in Nursing Roles" (*Amer. J. Sociol.* 66 (1961): 604–615). Corwin compares the self-concept of graduates from collegiate and diploma programs, and discusses their respective adjustments to the bureaucratized hospital setting.

2.   *Status (the Peck-Order):* The law of the peck-order is based on the behavior of the domestic hen, and is as follows: In a group of three hens: one will peck the two others; of these two, one will peck the other, who will peck no other. This pecking-order is a hierarchy that ensures an unequal distribution of privileges accompanied by a minimum amount of fighting. Peck-orders serving a similar purpose have been observed in other species of birds, in insects, and in many species of mammals including *Homo sapiens*. For example, the hierarchy of a gang resembles peck-order organization, and serves the same purpose: W. F. Whyte, *Street Corner Society* (Chicago: University of Chicago Press, 1943). No research to date contradicts the statement that rank and status differences are universal in human groups, even though the members of particular groups claim complete equality. Probably because of the heady notion that all members of a democracy are born to equal opportunity, there is considerable literature about socially organized inequalities.

The most significant attempts to explain inequality fall into three categories: biological differences, the need for cooperation, and the presence of conflicts.

The biological explanations do not satisfactorily account for the variations in human stratification systems. Studies about the relationship between performance level and innate ability cited at the end of this note support this statement. The main tenets of the theories stressing need for cooperation, the so-called functionalist explanation, are identified by Davis and Moore as:

(a) Tasks that need to be done in a society differ in importance, difficulty, and popularity.

(b) To see to it that tasks which may be either difficult and/or unpopular are performed, society rewards those who perform these tasks more highly than they reward those who perform less demanding and less vital tasks.

(c) In this manner society creates a system of differentially rewarding positions—the hierarchy.

Davis and Moore answer the question: "Who will do the important work?" by concluding that societies create hierarchies in order to get important work done (K. Davis and W. Moore, "Some Principles of Stratification," *Amer. Sociol. Rev.* 10 (1954): 242–249). A considerable body of literature has developed around the thesis summarized above, and Wrong's assessments of the strengths and weaknesses of the functional theory of stratification is recommended. (D. H. Wrong, "The Functional Theory of Stratification: Some Neglected Considerations," *Amer. Sociol. Rev.* 24 (1959): 772–782). The conflict-centered theory is most explicitly stated by Gumplowicz; and, in a sense, this body of theory is based on answers to the question: Who will do the dirty work? And the standard answer is: the out-group. L. Gumplowicz, *Grundiss der Sociologic* (Vienna: Manz, 1885). In western societies, as one might expect, the conflict theory has tended to develop in relation to the hypothesis that private property is the determinant of inequality. Marx was convinced that the abolition of private property would usher in equality but this notion has been tested and disproved. See A. Inkeles, "Social Stratification and Mobility in the Soviet Union" (*Amer. Sociol. Rev.* 15 (1950): 465–479).

Cooperation-centered theory focuses on answers to the question: Who does the important work? Conflict-centered theory focuses on answers to the question: Who does the dirty work? Both categories of work must be done, and in the doing of them the question of talent utilization becomes pertinent. The literature suggests that human talent is underutilized, particularly at lower levels in industrial societies. It seems probable that the physiological determinants of maximum ability are equally distributed throughout a society's hierarchy, but societies tend to resist higher mobilization of ability. Faris and Zetterberg suggest that levels of performance and innate capacity bear little relationship to each other (R. E. L. Faris, "Reflections on the Ability Dimension," *Amer. Sociol. Rev.* 26 (1961): 835–843 and H. L. Zitterberg, *Social Theory and Social Practice* [New York: Bedminster Press, 1962]).

The chief defect of socially stratified systems in industrial societies seems to be the low level of aspiration at lower, and numerically important, levels in the hierarchy. Studies about: Who goes to college: why and why not? show that innate ability, as measured by I. Q., is not the determining factor. In this country more than half of those with the most innate ability, top 10 percent, do not receive college educations according to Zetterberg (1962) and D. Wolfe, *American Resources of Specialized Talent* (New York: Harper & Row Publishers, 1954). In all western industrial societies, a study of recruitment to universities reveal a consistent under-representation of those with innate ability from lower socioeconomic levels in the society. Glass's estimate that if innate ability were the sole criterion 60 percent of the university's students would come from lower socioeconomic populations seems to be compatible with studies in other western industrial societies, including the United States. See D. V. Glass, *Education, Economy and Society* (New York: The Free Press, 1961), pp. 391–413.

3.   *Role:* Role and status sometimes are used as if they were synonomous, and the relationship between self and role is not always clearly delineated. A theoretical frame of reference developed by social psychologists is particularly valuable to those interested in studying roles, role theory. Role theory: clearly differentiates role and status; it shows the interrelatedness of role and status and points up the difference between self and role. In Chapter 6, Role Theory, *Handbook of Social Psychology,* G. Lindzey, ed. (Reading, Mass.: Addison-Wesley Publishing Company, Inc., 1954), Theodore Sarbin presents: role theory; the history of its development as an interdisciplinary theory; and the way it can be used to study human behavior at a relatively complex level. Sarbin's explanation of role theory is an excellent introduction to relevant theory. The basic conceptual units of role theory are: role, the unit of culture; status, the unit of society; and self, the unit of personality. Thus, role theory draws its variables from three disciplines: anthropology, sociology, and psychology.

4.   *The Hospital Patient:* There is a considerable literature about the hospital patient, and an excellent route into it is to read Parsons' classical analysis of the sick-role, and then to look at Coser's study of the hospital patient role which is, in my opinion, a classic: T. Parsons, *The Social System* (New York: The Free Press, 1951), Chapter X; and R. L. Coser, *Life in the Ward* (East Lansing, Mich.: Michigan University Press, 1962). The differences between the sick-role and the role of hospital patient are set forth in T. Parsons and R. Fox, "Illness, Therapy, and the Modern Urban Family," *J. Social Issues* 8, no. 4 (1952): 31–44. Probably the most useful book about the hospital patient, at least as far as those who work in hospitals are concerned, is Dr. Brown's book: E. L. Brown, *Newer Dimensions of Patient Care: Patients as People,* Part 3 (New York: Russell Sage Foundation, 1964). It not only provides the social concepts needed by hospital specialists who wish to recognize that patients are people but also it suggests ways in which this can be done.

5.   *The Patients Relationship to Professional Health Workers:* This subject is handled in considerable depth in Section VII "The Medical Setting: Hospital, Clinic and Office," in *Patients, Physicians, and Illness,* 3d ed., G. E. Jaco, ed. (New York: The Free Press, 1963), pp. 447–548.

PART THREE

Society and the Hospital:
The Roles and Relationships They Produce.

1. Society: The brief sketch of American society presented in this section is a product of observations of the changing society begun in 1947. The central question during these observations was: How is society reorganizing itself to confront the changing world? The most visible changes in the inanimate environment have been changes in technology, and as a consequence, I used what might be called an ecological approach. Ecologists recognize the interdependence of all living species, including plants and man, and their dependence, direct or indirect, on the inanimate environment. They conceptualize an interacting biotic and environmental system, and refer to it as an ecosystem.[6] L. Reid, *The Sociology of Nature,* rev. ed. (Baltimore: Penquin Books, Inc., 1962) provides an excellent example of this approach.

An ecological frame of reference is particularly valuable when the history of the development of institutions and practices are under consideration inasmuch as it permits us to raise such questions as: To what extent have the theories and practices of childbirth been influenced by the "delivery table," a piece of equipment initially designed to permit the male physician to grope around under a sheet, and deliver a baby without looking at the "private parts" of the mother? Lewis Mumford in *Technics and Civilization* (New York: Harcourt, Brace & World, Inc., 1934) uses this approach to raise interesting questions about society.

The tendency of organizations to increase in size, and families to decrease in size, commented on in my diagram of the launching-pad society (Fig. 6) is documented in the literature. (For documentation of this tendency in the family see note 3 in this section.) In 1963, the U.S. Bureau of the Census began to document the organization's tendency to increase in size. It showed that in 1958 72 percent of the 270,000 manufacturing companies in the country were single-unit companies employing fewer than twenty persons each, 6.5 percent of those employed in such organizations; whereas 0.13 percent were multiorganizations, employed 40 percent of the working force at the rate of 5000 or more workers each and, on average, operating 170 establishments each. According to the reports put out by this bureau, single-unit companies have decreased and multiorganizations have increased since 1958. Hawley (1950) calls multiorganizations "corporate" units, and provides an excellent description of them. The proliferation of large-scale groups of individuals with similar vested interests is pertinent to our understanding of changing American society. An analysis of this phenomenon is to be found in: E. E. Boulding, *The Organizational Revolution* (New York: Harper & Row, Publishers, 1953).

2. Family: There has been considerable controversy about the universal characteristics of the family. Murdock's definition of the family, and his identifi-

[6] This approach has been used both by sociologists and anthropologists. A. H. Hawley, *Human Ecology: A Theory of Community Structure* (New York: The Ronald Press Company, 1950); and J. Helm, "The Ecological Approach in Anthropology," *Amer. J. Sociol.* 67 (1962): 630–639.

cation of four primary functions which he claims are, in combination, universal, is supported by impressive evidence: G. P. Murdock, *Social Structure* (New York: Macmillan, 1949). An examination of information about families in 250 societies, led Murdock to conclude that the family is a social group consisting of husband, wife, and children with the following characteristics: sexual access permitted between adult members, reproduction occurs legitimately, responsibility to society for the care and upbringing of offspring, and an economic unit as far as consumption is concerned. Murdock's definition has been attacked, and what usually is objected to is his contention that the kinship group which performs the four family functions characterized by him invariably is a nuclear family composed of husband-father, wife-mother, son, and daughter. Levy, Spiro, Gough, and others have presented counter examples in which at least one of these four functions is performed by some other social group (M. E. Spiro, "Is the Family Universal?" *Amer. Anthro.* 56 (1954): 839–846; M. J. Levy and L. A. Fallers, "The Family: Some Comparative Considerations," *Amer. Anthro.* 61 (1959): 647–651; E. K. Gough, "The Nayars and the Definition of Marriage," *J. Roy. Anthro. Inst.* 89 (1959): 23–24). A proposal by Malinowski suggests one way in which arguments about the universal characteristic of the family might be settled. Rather than identifying a universal group as the family, Malinowski proposed an institutionalized norm, legitimate birth. Legitimate birth places the newborn in a position in the society, or subsociety, that is recognized by those members who have been socialized into it. And such a position regulates both the social relations of members with the newborn and the newborn's rights (B. Malinowski, "Parenthood—the Basis of Social Structure" in: V. F. Calverton and Schmalhausen, eds., *The New Generation* [New York: Macaulay Company, 1930] pp. 113–168).

Arguments against Malinowski's proposal center on illegitimacy rates. For example, at least eight Caribbean countries have illegitimacy rates of more than 60 percent (W. J. Goode, "Illegitimacy in the Caribbean Social Structures," *Amer. Sociol. Rev.* 25 (1960): 21–30). Goode argues that the high illegitimacy rates are not the result of an absence of legitimacy norms, and that they do not result because the subsociety sanctions illegitimate birth. According to Goode, they are the consequence of disorganization among lower class families. His argument is based on a careful examination of Caribbean courtship and marriage practices. In the vast majority of cases, the common-law marriages that produce an illegitimacy rate of more than 60 percent eventually are converted into "legitimate" marriages. This fact leads Goode to conclude that "legitimate" marriage is the preferred model. The fact that members of the subsociety in which this phenomenon occurs sanction common-law marriage and do not stigmatize the offspring of it suggests that this concept of illegitimacy is an alien one. According to Malinowski, a family exists when there is a "pater role" which determines the jural status, rights, and obligations of a child recognized as the pater's child, and when the pater is held responsible by other members of the society for the child's conduct. Malinowski's proposal seems to argue that the family is identified by members of this particular subculture (lower socioeconomic Caribbean) as one in which the female, with or without the benefit of "marriage lines," discharges the functions of the "pater role." The American

and the Caribbean Negro families usually are described as unstab!e and matrifocal. As far as the American scene is concerned, E. F. Frazier's book *The
Negro Family in the United States* (Chicago: University of Chicago Press,
1939) is a classical example of this approach, a judgment that was summed up
in the Moynihan Report.

R. T. Smith's analysis of quantitative data for British Guiana Negro communities supports my notion that the matrifocal family is an adaptive response
to a specific ecological niche (R. T. Smith, *The Negro Family in British Guiana*
[London: Routledge & Kegan Paul Ltd., 1956]).

3. The Nuclear Family: When father, mother, and child form a recognizable
unit in society, this unit is referred to as the nuclear family. This family system
is organized around a husband-wife axis, capable of discharging family functions
in a number of different ways. These possibilities are referred to in the literature
as "typologies," and the nuclear family is "typed" according to who makes
decisions about what and according to who does whatever is required to discharge family functions. Herbst's study of urban Australian families, Bott's
study of London families, and Wolfe's study of the family as a power system
combine the logical possibilities in somewhat different ways (P. G. Herbst, "The
Measurement of Family Relationships," *Hum. Relat.* 5 (1952): 3–35; E. Bott,
Family and Social Network [London: Tavistock Publishers, 1957]; D. Wolfe,
"Power and Authority in the Family" in *Studies in Social Power,* D. Cartwright,
ed. [Ann Arbor: University of Michigan Press, 1959], pp. 99–117). In American society, nuclear families break down when there are dynamic changes in the
balance of power within the family system, and Koos's longditudinal study of
sixty-two low income, New York families shows the dynamics of this process
(E. L. Koos, *Families in Trouble* [New York: King's Crown Press, 1946]). It
also shows why matrifocal family systems which are productive adjustments to
a specific ecological niche frequently are thought of as "broken families."

4. Kinship Systems: The kinship system most frequently encountered in American society is bilateral: one that includes two blood lines, those of both biological father and biological mother. Murdock and Freeman are recommended
as sources of information about kinship systems (G. P. Murdock, "Cognatic
Forms of Social Organization," in *Social Structure in South East Asia,* G. P.
Murdock, ed. [Chicago: Quadrangle Books, 1960] and J. D. Freeman, "On the
Concept of Kindred," *J. Roy Anthro. Inst.* 91 (1961): 192–220).

*5. Nuclear Families That Have Detached Themselves from Bilateral Kinship
Systems:* The literature on the emergence of bilateral kinship systems and the
partial detachment of the nuclear family from it centers on the question of
whether or not the phenomena are products of industrialization. Ogburn,
Burgess, and Parsons suggest that they are (E. W. Burgess, "The Family as a
Unity of Interacting Personalities," *The Family* 7 (1926): 3–9; W. F. Ogburn,
"The Changing Family," *Publ. Amer. Sociol. Soc.* 23 (1928): 124–133; and
T. Parsons, "The Kinship Systems of the Contemporary United States," *Amer.
Anthro.* 45 (1943): 22–28). Historical evidence confirms the presence of these

phenomena prior to the Industrial Revolution. J. E. A. Jolliffe, *Prefeudal England: The Jutes* (London: Oxford University Press, 1959). In addition, there is evidence that some of the most primitive hunting-gathering cultures are organized around detached nuclear families (See M. F. Nimkoff, and R. Middleton, "Types of Family and Types of Economy," *Amer. J. Sociol.* 66 (1960): 215–225).

The evidence suggests that industrialization is not necessary to produce bilateral kinship systems and detached nuclear families, but that it is capable of changing otherwise organized kinship and family systems in this direction. Greenfield's argument is most succinct: he showed that certain features of industrialization, rather than industrialization per se, are associated with these changes (S. Greenfield, "Industrialization and the Family in Sociological Theory," *Amer. J. Sociol.* 67 (1961): 312–322). The way in which these modifications emerge is described by Ross and Dore (R. P. Dore, *City Life in Japan* [Berkeley: University of California Press, 1958] and A. D. Ross, *The Hindu Family in its Urban Setting* [Toronto: University of Toronto Press, 1962]).

My own description of the mobile nuclear family, which I refer to as the launching-pad family, is an over-simplification designed to draw attention to "kindred" groups that no longer exercise authority over the nuclear family. However, it was my observation that parents continue to support the nuclear families of their own offspring, subsidizing the income of married children, and helping during childbirth and other family crises. Mutually supportive behavior between adult siblings also can be observed. Reiss confirms these observations, and suggests that the mobility of the nuclear family merely reduces the effective range of extended kinship systems (P. J. Reiss, "The Extended Kinship System: Correlates of and Attitudes on Frequency of Interaction," *Mar. Fam. Living* 24 (1962): 333–339).

6. *The Cracker Culture:* The subculture described in this chapter is similar in many ways to the "frontier" model described by Pearsall in "Cultures of the American South," *Anthro. Quart.* 39, no. 2 (1966): 128–141. It began in the same way and in the same geographical areas. Unlike Pearsall's frontier culture, it shows the influence of the yeoman farmers: "the 'Plain Folk of the Old South' whose Calvanistic tradition mixed with that of the frontier" (Pearsall 1966: 137). I first became interested in what Pearsall refers to as the "cultural mix" of the South in 1947 when I began to compare the residue of the plantation culture in one county in Virginia with the culture of an isolated community "The Free State" in the foothills of the Blue Ridge mountains. The latter was a frontier culture similar to the one described by Pearsall. In 1952 I moved to Florida, and began to examine a postfrontier type county that was referred to by residents as "typical Cracker." My description of the "Cracker" culture was formalized in 1959, and used to provide nurses from other parts of the United States with some understanding of patients who had been reared in the Florida Cracker culture. On a number of occasions it has been read, and my conclusions validated, by Floridians who grew up in the culture that I have attempted to describe.

7. *Leisure Value Systems:* Theory relevant to the concept developed here was proposed first by Thorstan Veblen in *The Theory of the Leisure Class: An Economic Study of Institutions* (New York: The Modern Library, 1934). His conclusion was that when mobility increased and material level rose, as it dramatically has done in industrial societies since the beginning of the Industrial Revolution, traditional value systems tend to be replaced by value systems modeled on the way in which those at superior economic levels in the society used available money and time to amuse themselves. During the nineteenth century and the early part of the present century, considerable energy was expended on the task of "edifying" the "poor"—attempts to impose bourgeois values of thrift, austerity, and production on those at lower socioeconomic levels in the society. Failure to do so resulted in the hypothesis that the form taken by leisure activities in industrial societies is a product of the need to compensate for the deprivations and constraints of the work situation. During the past fifteen years, considerable research energy has been devoted to disproving this hypothesis, and the alternate one that leisure activities reflect the direction and level of work performance. Dumazedier offers convincing arguments as far as the American scene is concerned. J. Dumazedier, *Towards a Society of Leisure* (New York: The Free Press, 1967). Two European observers of the relationship between leisure and consumer behavior confirm Veblen's thesis and support Dumazedier's contentions. In A. Pizzorono, "Accumulation, Loisirs et Rapports de Classe," *Esprit* (June 1959), Pizzorono suggests that the bourgeois values that were "wished onto" the working class were incompatible with its situation in industrial societies, and that leisure values developed as a counter system. F. Alberoni in *Consumi e Societa* (Bologna: Il Mullno, 1959) makes the same point, but focuses on a significant change in frame of reference: that rising income and increased mobility permit lower class man to look beyond the local, bourgeois-dominated community as a reference for style of life. Obviously, this tendency increases as mass media makes what we might call the national life style increasingly visible to those at lower socioeconomic levels in the society. Veblen's insight and the work of Pizzorono and Alberoni encourage us to look in a new way at our changing society. For example, observers of the society sometimes wonder why the power and authority of capital and management are not challenged; they also wonder why those at lower socioeconomic levels direct their attention toward amusement rather than toward seeing to it that the rewards within the society are redistributed. It also suggests that leisure is patterned in such a way as to provide meaning in everyday life. Crozier and Touraine support the latter suggestion (M. Crozier, "Les Mondes des Employés de Bureau," *Le Seuil* (Paris 1965); and A. Touraine, "Sociologie de l'Action." *Le Seuil* [Paris 1966]). E. Goffman, in *Presentation of Self in Everyday Life* (New York: Doubleday & Company, Inc., 1959) seems to agree.